STRENGTH AND
CONDITIONING FOR TRIATHLON

MARK JARVIS

STRENGTH AND CONDITIONING FOR TRIATHLON

The 4th Discipline

BLOOMSBURY

LONDON · NEW DELHI · NEW YORK · SYDNEY

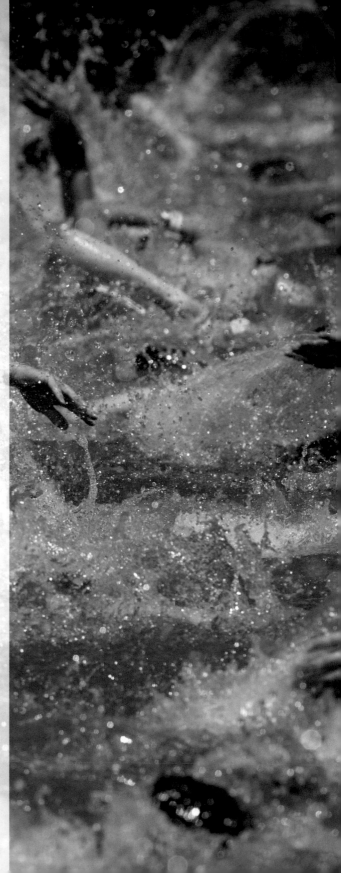

Published by Bloomsbury Publishing Plc
50 Bedford Square
London WC1B 3DP
www.bloomsbury.com

First edition 2013
Copyright © 2013 Mark Jarvis

ISBN (print): 978 1 4081 7211 7
ISBN (Epub): 978 1 4081 8141 6
ISBN (EPDF): 978 1 4081 7960 4

A CIP catalogue record for this book is available from the British Library.

Acknowledgements
Cover photograph © Getty Images
Inside photographs: All images courtesy of Grant Pritchard with the exception of the following: This page, pp.1, 2, 8, 10, 11, 14, 17, 18, 20–21, 22, 24, 26, 27, 33, 42, 44–45, 48, 54, 56–57, 59, 60, 63, 64–65, 66, 73, 79, 82–83, 84, 87, 89, 92, 95, 96, 98, 110–111, 112, 137, 154, 155, 156, 169, 174, 182 © Shutterstock images
p. 182 © Maxisport/Shutterstock and p. 56–57 © Martin Good/Shutterstock
Designer: James Watson
Illustrations by David Gardner
Commissioning Editor: Kirsty Schaper
Editor: Sarah Cole

This book is produced using paper that is made from wood grown in managed, sustainable forests. It is natural, renewable and recyclable. The logging and manufacturing processes conform to the environmental regulations of the country of origin.

Typeset in Meta Plus by seagulls.net

Printed and bound in China by C&C Offset Printing Co

10 9 8 7 6 5 4 3 2 1

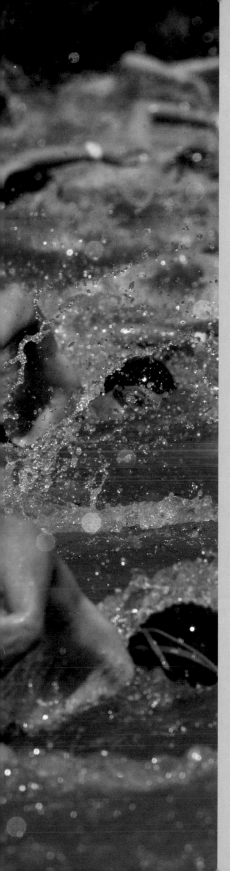

contents

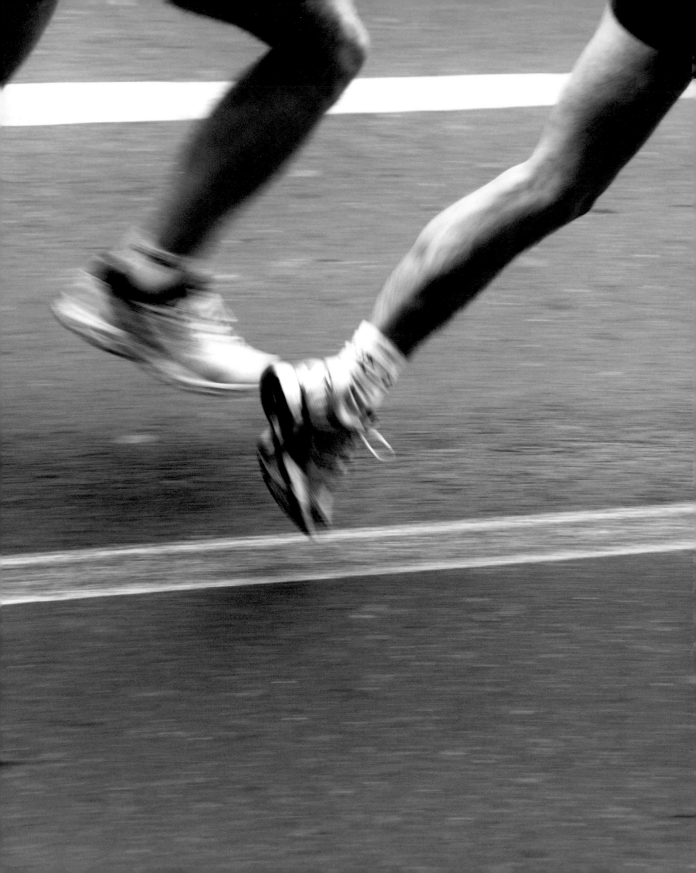

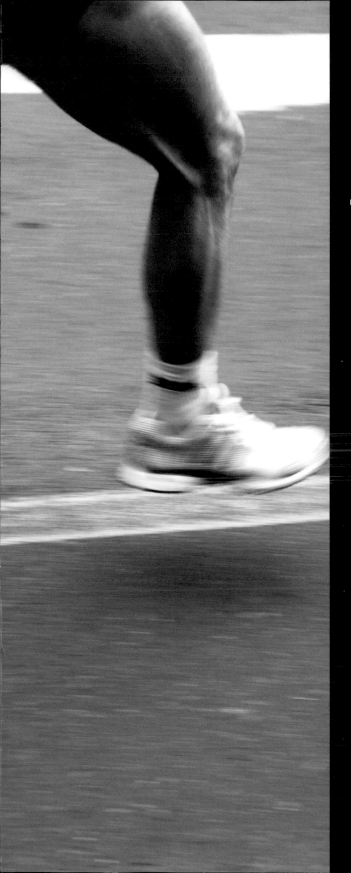

part 1

training concepts

001
what is strength and conditioning?

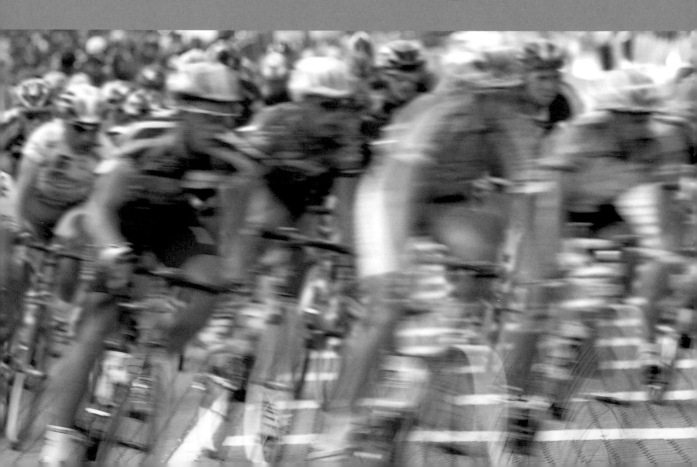

1.1 Introduction

Ask any coach worth their salt if they use strength and conditioning (S&C) and chances are they will hurriedly agree and extol its importance. However getting them to define exactly what this means tends to draw a vague or at best narrow answer. This is not entirely surprising though. The term 'strength and conditioning' has only really emerged in the UK in the past decade. Even the words themselves can cause some confusion. What do we mean by strength? What exactly is conditioning? Clearly it is worth exploring the terminology properly before we go any further.

Possibly the best sound bite definition for S&C is: 'The physical preparation of athletes towards enhancing sports performance and reducing injury.' Essentially this means that S&C can encompass all forms of physical training outside of technical and tactical work. Consequently almost all triathlon training could technically be classified as S&C! In reality though the swim, bike and run components of training are classified as 'normal training', while S&C refers to any derivates of the three disciplines as well as any other physical work. Perhaps the French say it best with their term 'Preparateur physique'!

1.2 What is strength?

Perhaps the most confusing element of S&C is the 'S'. The word 'strength' conjures images of muscle-bound men lifting huge barbells in macho gyms. Clearly this is not the image of the podium triathlete. A more useful way of looking at strength is the production or control of force. As a result strength can come in many forms.

Absolute strength

This describes most people's immediate thoughts regarding strength. Simply put, this refers to the

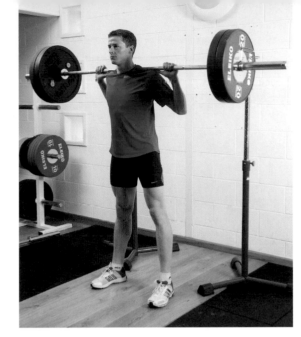

Figure 1.1a Athlete A – 100kg

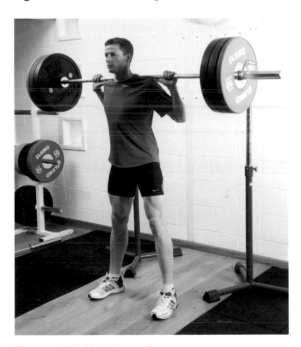

Figure 1.1b Athlete B – 120kg

greatest amount of total force an individual can generate. For example, if athlete A can lift a barbell weighing 100kg and athlete B can lift 120kg, athlete B has greater absolute strength. In reality this has little direct relevance to triathlon performance. The most obvious use of this quality comes during cycling when the ability to apply large forces through the crank will be a key determinant of cycling speed. This becomes especially important during sprints and flat sections of the race. Absolute strength also has a role to play as a building block to other strength qualities. Even if we are not using this quality directly, having a 'strength reserve' means that we are working at a lower percentage of our maximum and so performance is less physically stressful and more controlled.

Relative strength

Our own body weight must be taken into consideration in relative strength. This is clearly crucial in triathlon as the essence of the sport is to transport one's own body around a course! Let's take the previous example of athletes A and B. If we now consider that athlete A weighs 70kg and athlete B weighs 90kg, and we divide their lifts by their body weight we can see that athlete A is able to lift 1.4 times body weight whereas athlete B is only lifting 1.3 times. Therefore athlete A actually has the superior relative strength despite lifting a lighter bar. Of course it is possible to improve both our absolute and relative strength at the same time if we get stronger and remain at the same weight (more on this below). Interestingly we can also improve our relative strength by losing weight (i.e. fat) without actually getting stronger.

Relative strength is particularly important for the run and during hill climbs. The athlete with a low body weight but the ability to produce strong running and powerful hill climbs will be hard to beat.

Postural strength

This may be the element of strength most removed from the tradition view but it is critical to the triathlete. Picture the swimmer whose technique slowly becomes rougher and rougher as fatigue sets in. Imagine the cyclist who sprints to take a rival, but the bike rocks from side to side as they struggle to control the power their legs are generating. Or perhaps you can relate to the poor runner who slumps forward as if battling a hurricane while shuffling their feet more like an ice skater than an athlete. All of these lack postural strength and are destined never to fulfil their true athletic potential. When we lack postural strength we lose mechanical efficiency. Think how different most people's running technique looks from textbook images. Now imagine training and competing on a bike that was as inefficient. Triathletes ignore efficiency at their peril!

So, if it is so important, why do so many ignore postural strength? The answer may lie in the fact that making improvements is not always a simplistic process. Postural strength is a combination of muscle strength and motor coordination. For example, it is too simplistic to think that doing some abdominal exercises on the floor will automatically lead to better trunk control in the pool. Similarly a triathlete will always struggle to perform drills properly and to make technical progress if their muscles are simply too weak to make the movements that they are being asked to produce. The key to success is in combining these two factors and evaluating where the weak link lies.

Explosive strength

At the opposite end of the spectrum is explosive strength, or power, which is the sexy part of strength training. Particularly in the shorter distances, power makes all the difference. Who has the kick at the end of the race, who can break away in a sprint or a hill climb? Interestingly power data from Tour de France cyclists show that for many periods of the race the riders work at power

Table 1.1	Strength factors in swim, bike and run		
	Swim	**Bike**	**Run**
Absolute strength	*	**	*
Relative strength	**	***	**
Postural strength	***	*	***
Explosive strength	*	***	**
Reactive strength	*	*	***

outputs that most of us are capable of sustaining. However it is during the brief but critical bursts that these riders show their true class with impressive displays of pure explosive power. If we look to the track we see similar trends. Most 5,000-metre and 10,000-metre races at the world-class level involve relatively steady laps for most of the race. Despite maintaining a hugely impressive tempo, the bell signals an incredible sprint to the finish with top male runners often having to put in final laps in the region of 52 seconds in order to claim gold.

Reactive strength

Also known as elastic strength, reactive strength is critical to the way we run. This is explained in detail in chapter 6. However in simple terms efficient runners are able to use the elastic properties of tendons and muscles to store and reuse so-called elastic energy. This can account for around half of the energy production during running. So when you see high-class distance runners effortlessly gliding along the ground it is no illusion!

Training for improvements in reactive strength involves a combination of physical and technical changes. While some changes in the body are

important, it is also necessary to put the body in the right positions to utilise this. Again this is discussed in much greater detail later on.

Table 1.1 gives a guide as to how each of these strength qualities relates to the three triathlon disciplines.

Already it is clear that there is more to strength than many people imagine ... and we have still only dealt with half of the S&C.

1.3 What is conditioning?

The answer to this question depends very much on which sport conditioning is being applied to. In team sports, for example, this may be used to describe the metabolic training – or 'fitness' in everyday terms. However in triathlon terms it is more likely to mean getting muscles up to the task of coping with the demands made of training. In this sense it could be regarded as primarily being injury prevention work or perhaps even another type of strength.

So why do we need to do this on top of normal training? Often we may identify a mechanical issue within the body which either causes trouble now or is likely to in the future. This may be a result of a prior injury or commonly an adaptation in our body to the unnatural amounts of time most of us spend sitting down. The problem here is that each time we swim, ride or run the poor mechanics are rehearsed further and become ever more strongly ingrained. Therefore it is necessary to intervene with conditioning exercises, which give the athlete the opportunity to rehearse and learn the correct movement. Additionally exercises may be included to strengthen, stretch or mobilise areas that are causing the problem.

A classic example of this occurs in the shoulder of the swimmer. The shoulder, and all of the body, has some muscles that are intended for controlling movement (stabilisers) and others that are made for producing movement (prime movers). Commonly the stabilisers become weak and under active while the prime movers start to take over as stabilisers (more on this in chapter 3). This could reasonably be described as square pegs in round holes. As a result the shoulder becomes less stable and movements around the joint become less smooth than they should be. It can be surprising how small deviations in movement control can be catastrophic. However when you consider that even a relatively short swim session may involve performing the same action well in excess of 1,000 times it is easy to see that microscopic levels of wear and tear can add up.

As you can imagine, the process of identifying and addressing these issues can be quite complex. To be fully effective a conditioning programme requires the same level of insight into the mechanics of the body (biomechanics) that is possessed by a bike mechanic. In recent years a process known as a 'functional movement screen' has been employed to assess mechanics and movement. Triathletes have also tended to use

rather haphazard conditioning exercises, which they have collected along the way from friends, magazines or sneakily observed someone else in the gym doing. This scattergun type of approach is most likely to be at best inefficient and at worst ineffective. One of the key aims of this book is to enable the reader to understand their own conditioning needs (yourself or a client) and to address them as efficiently and effectively as possible. This is dealt with in depth in chapter 3.

1.4 Practical S&C

Having explored exactly what we mean by the term S&C it is worth discussing exactly what strength and conditioning looks like in real life.

What are the tools of S&C?

Given that we are thinking of S&C as 'physical preparation' it should come as no surprise that there is no limitation as to what can be included in an S&C session. S&C coaches can be considered the magpies of sports science in that they take their tools from myriad sources. These will include track and field, Olympic lifting, power lifting, physiotherapy and even yoga. Over the past decade the profession has evolved to the extent that S&C coaches have also developed their own tools, which are distinct from any of these other original

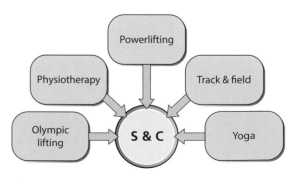

Figure 1.2 S&C influences

influences. The only limit comes from the imagination of the coach. Subsequently having access to an exclusive gym, or any gym at all for that matter, is no barrier. In fact the lack of a gym may even promote more creative and individualised sessions rather than simply defaulting to standard exercises, which the gym may lend itself to.

What might a typical session involve?

When it comes to triathlon S&C there really are no rules regarding exactly how a session may look. Triathlon is three sports rolled into one, which makes for a wide variety of physiques, strengths and weaknesses, and physical attributes of those who take part. Combine these with differing ages, genders and levels of training experience and clearly a one-size-fits-all approach is never going to be effective. Therefore there are no 'rules' regarding where a session should occur, how long it should take or what should go into it. If that sounds as if there is no system involved rest assured that there are still key principles that must be adhered to if good and consistent progress is to be made. Namely, these are overload, progression, variety/variation and specificity.

1.5 Principles of training

The principles of training are as simple as they are fundamental. However it is amazing how often these are ignored in training programmes, particularly by triathletes.

Overload

For this the exercises must stress the athlete to a greater degree than they usually experience. When the body is subjected to an appropriate level of overload there will be an initial suppression followed by a supercompensation. This means that the body will repair itself in order to be better

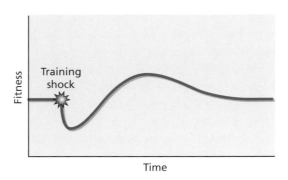

Figure 1.3 Principle of supercompensation

prepared for future challenges. This is the essence of all training. If there is not enough overload then the body simply won't adapt. Essentially this is because the training has been too easy. If the overload is too great the body will either fail to recover or will potentially get injured. For example, if a novice athlete tried to copy the training session of an experienced trainer the level of overload is likely to be too great and the athlete will suffer as a result. This process of a dip in fitness followed by recovery is illustrated in figure 1.3.

If we really have a good understanding of our training and what we are trying to achieve we can be very precise in selecting which element of performance we overload. For example, if we wish to overload our speed and reactive strength we may use some sprints in training. Alternatively we may wish to overload our skill and technical development in the pool and use drills to achieve this.

Progression

Progression is arguably the most commonly ignored principle by triathletes. I have met countless triathletes who will tell me they do some strength and conditioning. They will then go on to describe a routine that they have put together, which sounds reasonably appropriate. It is only when they then go on to say that they have been performing exactly the same routine for the past three seasons that the flaw in their plan is exposed! While their routine may have initially produced some gains they will very quickly have plateaued and ceased to make any further progress. By failing to make any progression the overload is reduced or removed as the body becomes too comfortable with the session. This seems to go against all common sense. It seems unthinkable that any triathlete would consider performing exactly the same swim, bike and running sessions week after week and still expect to make progress. Yet for some reason this sensible logic seems to escape many athletes when it comes to their S&C. In reality this is most likely to come from a lack of awareness of how much better they could be and frequently the athlete simply doesn't know how to progress the session. This book will guide you in how to take all aspects of S&C from introductory level to elite. It is worth noting that progression in some areas is not always

required. For example, flexibility is a quality that we require only adequate levels of, as opposed to more always being better. In this situation we work to attain the required standard and then shift our attention to other areas. The joy of multi-discipline sports is that there is *always* something else to work on. Other qualities such as speed will always have a place in the programme. I am yet to discover the athlete who wouldn't want any more speed.

Variety or variation

This also often suffers from a lack of understanding of how to take a programme forward, and will potentially result in staleness and stagnation. Consider the following example:

Chris decided that he wanted to improve his upper body strength and so started to include some press-ups in his training. Having not done any upper body training other than swimming this gave him the overload he needed. When he started

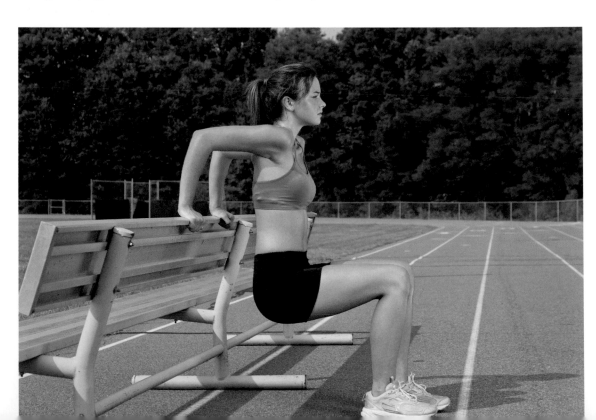

he found 4 sets of 10 press-ups pretty tough. After a few sessions this became easier and so he gradually added a few more repetitions until he was able to perform 4 sets of 20 press-ups. Chris was really pleased with this progress and so continued to try to increase the number of press-ups he did in each set. Frustratingly though he couldn't seem to get beyond 20. This was inevitable as sooner or later we reach a limit in a given exercise. The answer to Chris's problem lies in variation. By changing the nature of the exercise he will give his body a new stimulus. Obviously this must have some relevance to the previous exercise in order to build on previous gains. Suitable examples might be slightly different types of press-up (such as with a weight on his back) or a similar dumb-bell exercise. By using this variety Chris will have a good chance of getting over his plateau and may find that if he returns to his press-ups in a few weeks he may be able to move beyond his 20-repetition sticking point.

Specificity

Finally we come to specificity. This is possibly the concept that causes the most confusion among coaches. The phrase 'sports specific' has often been misinterpreted as meaning that the event itself is mimicked with weights. For example, attempting to perform a replication of the swimming stroke with small weights in each hand. This is not only a very ineffective practice but may also actually lead to a decrease in performance. While the movements may look similar to the eye, what happens in the body is very different. The motor pattern (message from the brain to the muscles) will be very different as the speed and control involved in the movement will be hugely different due to the weight. The fact that the action is similar to that of the sport may actually lead to a phenomenon known as 'negative transfer'. This means that the finely tuned skill becomes 'polluted'.

Perhaps a more useful phrase could be 'sports relevant'. This simply reflects the fact that qualities that are related to the event are trained. This may mean that an exercise is relevant as it closely mimics (or overloads) the forces involved in the event and has some degree of mechanical relevance. A good example can be seen in the back squat exercise when used to improve cycling power. Even though the movement obviously differs from the action of cycling it still uses the hips, knees and ankles in a synchronised way. The exercise is useful as it forces you to push harder than you would even up a steep hill (therefore you have overload as well as specificity). However if you were simply to do leg curls you are unlikely to gain any benefit as the movement is too far removed from the action of cycling.

1.6 Science of S&C

Since the 1960s when Eastern Bloc researchers started taking a serious interest in strength training and performance enhancement much has been studied and written on the subject. Rather than repeat what has gone before the focus of this section is to give interested athletes an insight into why training programmes look like they do and to assist coaches in deepening their understanding of S&C.

Movement versus muscles

One of the things that most notably separates an S&C programme from the type of session most people perform in the gym is the type of exercises used. This has changed slightly in recent years as S&C has become more fashionable. However there is still a predominance of resistance machines and single-joint exercises in health club gyms. It is often said that S&C involves the training of movements, not muscles. This makes perfect sense as it reflects the way in which the body works. Although certain muscle groups may dominate a movement it is impossible to isolate a single muscle voluntarily. When we move, our brains brilliantly coordinate a synchronised response among numerous muscles, which all play a different role throughout the movement. Sometimes they are required to contract to produce force, within milliseconds their role may then switch to relaxation to allow another muscle to produce a smooth movement. Therefore to train effectively we need to train 'the whole orchestra' together so as not to upset the balance. It is highly misguided to assume that working on one muscle in an isolated way will then result in a positive change to a different and complex movement pattern.

Consider the following example: during the swim stroke (front crawl) our pecs (the chest) are used to pull the arm from extended out in front of us, down towards the hip. If we take this information away with us down to the local gym and jump on to the pec dec machine we are doomed to failure (as well as potentially increasing our risk of shoulder injury and worsening our technique). What we have missed is that although the pecs are important they are assisted by the lats, the serratus anterior and the abdominals to name but a few. By not involving these key players we will never achieve the result we want – even if we do look better in trunks now! A more effective strategy would be to use an exercise such as the pull-up. This will involve all of the aforementioned muscles in a way that is relevant, although not identical, to the action we are trying to improve.

The movement that is most frequently talked about in S&C is known as the triple extension. This describes a simultaneous extension of the hips, knees and ankles. There are very few sporting actions that do not involve a triple extension in some form. Think of how all three joints work together during the pedal stroke or during the running cycle. Swimming may be a rare

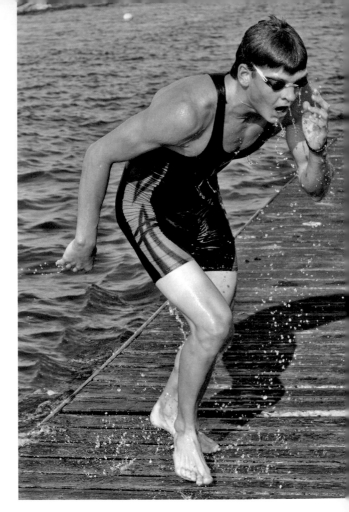

exception to this rule, although it is still featured in actions such as the dive into the water and the push-off-the-wall during the turn. It is because of the significance of this that exercises such as squats and lunges are so popular for strength gains and that jumping activities are used to develop speed and power in the triple extension.

What happens when we train?
One of the biggest barriers to starting an S&C programme for many triathletes is a lack of understanding regarding what will happen to their bodies. Therefore it is important to examine this to remove fears, as well as enable more precise coaching and programming to get the best possible gains.

By far the most common objection to a strength training programme is 'I don't want to do weights because I don't want to get big.' Sadly this comes from the association many people still have with weight training and bodybuilding. Fortunately the view is highly misguided and, provided they work to an appropriate programme, there should be no fears around gaining unwanted bulky muscles.

This news may leave some people scratching their heads. If my muscles don't get bigger, how can they get stronger? The answer, at least in part, lies in what is known as neural adaptations. In simple terms this refers to the ability of our nervous system to make the muscles do what we want. The average untrained individual is actually pretty poor at this. That may be the reason that most of the initial strength gains from a strength-training programme are thought to come from these neural adaptations.

But what exactly changes? There are four main aspects that we are able to affect with training:

- The signals to our muscles to move come in very rapid pulses rather than a constant stimulus. When we train these pulses occur much more rapidly and so muscles are told to move many more times per second than previously (this is known as rate coding). This results in more force or speed being produced.

- Each nerve that enters a muscle will control a certain number of muscle fibres – this is called a motor unit. If the nerve 'fires' then all of its muscle fibres will contract. Surprisingly the average person is able to activate only 30–40 per cent of their motor units even when highly motivated. With training this number can increase dramatically.

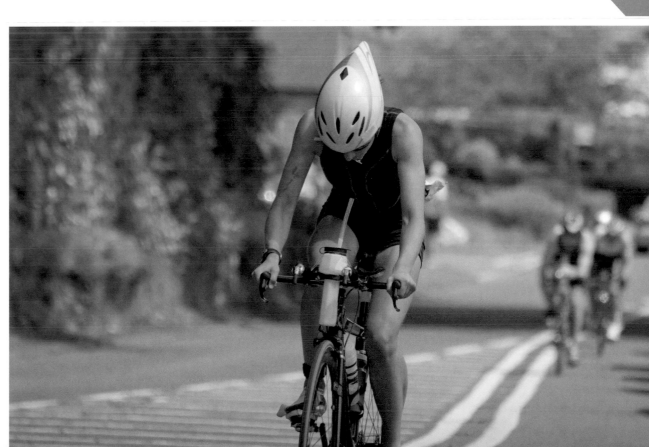

- As we become more used to exerting ourselves our nervous system is also better able to synchronise the signals to the muscles. Imagine a tug-of-war team. With no training all the members pull at different times and so they are not particularly effective. With training all of the signals occur closely together and so the resulting force created is a sum of these pulls.

- Finally our coordination between muscles becomes much better. This means that the pattern of when to contract and when to relax is much better. This makes for much more efficient movement.

These neural adaptations are highly significant. However it would be dishonest to suggest that there are no adaptations in the muscle, including tissue growth. This concept may scare many endurance athletes, but this need not be the case. There are two types of muscle growth (hypertrophy) that can happen following strength training: sarcoplasmic and myofibrillar. Sarcoplasmic hypertrophy results in more fluid within the muscle, giving it the 'pumped' look (*see* figure 1.4). Not surprisingly this occurs following bodybuilding-type programmes. Myofibrillar hypertrophy means that more myofibrils (the bits that contract and do the work) are packed into a

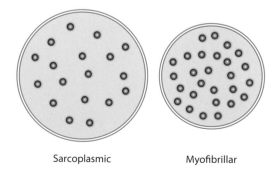

Sarcoplasmic   Myofibrillar

Figure 1.4 Types of hypertrophy

given space. Therefore it is possible to have muscle growth without growing big muscles!

Types of muscle contraction

Muscles work to produce movement by contracting (shortening) and moving the bones they are attached to via tendons. Three types of contraction are generally discussed:

- Concentric contraction occurs when the athlete tenses a muscle and it results in shortening.

- Eccentric contraction involves tensing the muscle but it still lengthens. An example of this would be when lowering a weight while still controlling it.

- Isometric contraction involves the muscle doing work but no movement occurring. A good example of this occurs at the trunk while swimming, when the muscles work to prevent unwanted movement occurring and help to maintain technique.

All of this may seem academic and somewhat irrelevant. However when we come to putting together training plans it is important to understand the types of contraction used in a particular movement so that we can train them with much greater specificity.

In a similar vein muscles are also considered to have primary functions for which they are best suited. On a simple level we can describe muscles as deep or superficial. Generally deep muscles provide postural control. These are mechanically suitable for providing stability to joints and can hold isometric contractions for a long period. On the other hand superficial muscles are ideal for producing movement. Many injuries and movement problems occur as a result of muscles acting in a manner that does not suit their purpose. A classic example of this is around the shoulder. If the muscles of the rotator cuff are weak then the superficial muscles take over and problems such as poor control and excessive tightness frequently occur.

Recovery

As we have already seen from figure 1.3, the essence of training is that we break ourselves down through training and then recover to a greater level than before. Therefore the recovery from training, rather than training itself, is what makes us fitter, stronger, faster, etc. Consequently it comes as no surprise that in recent years recovery has become a hot topic. It is now not only fashionable but commonplace to see athletes in ice baths, wearing skin tight compression garments and guzzling all manner of recovery drinks. The purpose of all these interventions is to accelerate recovery. Theoretically this will then allow the athlete to train more frequently (*see* figure 1.5).

However more recently an opposing theory has emerged, which suggests that if we use recovery methods to reduce the impact of the training shock we may in turn blunt the training response. Clearly this is not what we want to see. Therefore it may be best to save some of these recovery interventions for

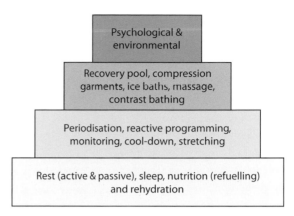

Figure 1.6 The recovery pyramid (Jarvis and Grantham)
www.dedicatedtofitness.com.au/images/Recovery.pdf

the competitive season when our aim is to recover from the exertions of competition and stay fresh.

The recovery methods chosen by athletes are also a contentious issue. If you were to ask the average triathlete what they do for recovery you will typically be greeted with a response featuring 'extreme interventions' such as ice baths and compression garments. However, while these tools may have their place, perhaps they should be regarded as the icing rather than the cake. A more balanced approach to recovery is described by the recovery pyramid (*see* figure 1.6)

This concept suggests that getting 'the basics' right first should be the priority rather than some of the sexier interventions. It is commonplace, even for elite athletes, to finish training and jump straight into an ice bath, dry down and slip into compression tights before booking in for an afternoon massage. However if the same athlete ignores the benefits of refuelling and rehydrating as soon as possible and getting off their feet for some rest, then all of their other efforts will be in vain. It may not seem very exciting, but when your Mum told you to get a hot meal and a good night's sleep she may have just given you the ultimate recovery protocol!

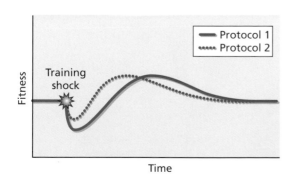

Figure 1.5 Theoretical accelerated recovery curve

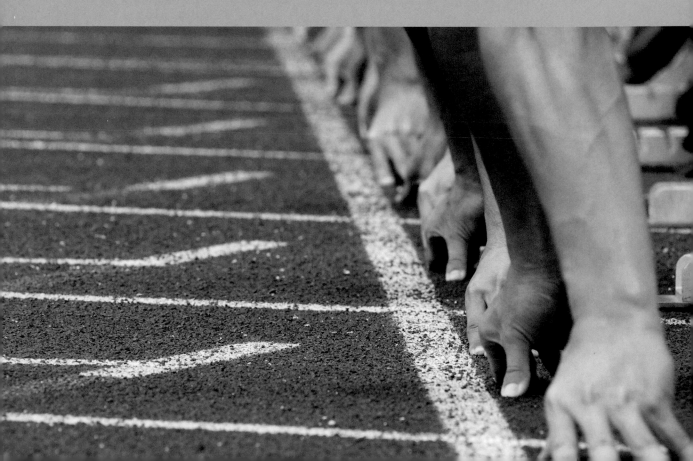

002
strength and conditioning for endurance sports

2.1 Introduction

As a strength and conditioning coach I can vouch for the fact that convincing coaches and athletes from endurance sports that they will benefit from strength training can be a tough task. This may not be entirely surprising as much of the scientific evidence to support this has emerged only in recent years. Endurance sport is immersed in a tradition of exclusively working on the metabolic side of fitness rather than strength qualities and movement efficiency. Therefore the S&C coach is faced with the daunting task of trying to change an entire culture.

It could be argued that the term 'endurance sport' itself is rather misleading. Clearly endurance is required, but the winner is still the one who completes the course fastest! If it were truly an endurance sport then the aim would be to see who can keep going at a standard pace the longest.

2.2 Strength versus endurance – is there a conflict?

Historically it has been believed that strength training and endurance training exist in opposition and that the two cannot sit side by side without compromising both. This is known as concurrent training. There is actually some basis for this belief. However in recent years our understanding of the mechanisms behind strength gains and endurance gains has increased, and by manipulating the timing of training and nutrition we can control these factors to our benefit. It should also be remembered that we have a broad definition of strength with regard to triathlon training and performance. Most of the concerns regarding concurrent training relate to maximal strength training. However this is a very small or non-existent component of the training we are discussing. The physical adaptations that produce gains in postural strength, reactive strength, etc. are largely seen in the nervous system

and so can be performed with no compromise or adverse effects.

However when we are working on developing a more traditional view of strength we must be aware of what is happening when we perform a strength session and when we perform an endurance session. When taking part in swim, bike and running sessions glycogen (the form carbohydrate takes in the body) is commonly used as an energy source. Therefore when we finish a session glycogen is generally low. This, along with other energy markers in the body such as levels of AMP, act as the catalyst for our body to start making the physical changes that will result in us getting fitter. Adenosine Monophosphate is a 'normal' energy molecule known as ATP and has 3 'energy units'. During exercise these are broken down until only one remains, forming AMP. Clearly then we want our bodies to stay in this state as long as possible in order to maximise our training gains.

On the other hand, the triggers our body needs to start adapting to strength training are almost exactly the opposite to the endurance triggers. High levels of glycogen, large intakes of protein (particularly essential amino acids such as leucine) and low levels of AMP will all promote the activation of a biochemical known as mTOR – a messenger in the body which signals for us to start synthesising protein for building/repairing muscle. When we achieve this state our bodies start to use the protein we have consumed to build more densely packed, powerful muscles. This state can last for up to 48 hours but will be 'switched off' if we reverse it with endurance training.

If we use this information smartly we can plan our training sessions to get the maximum benefit from both forms of training. To do this we need to follow a few simple rules:

- Keep strength and endurance sessions as far apart as possible. Going straight from one session to another is never going to be a particularly effective strategy. Where possible they should be placed either on different days or at least at opposite ends of the day. This will allow the body to stay in the 'endurance adaptation' and 'strength adaptation' state for as long as possible before being switched off.

- Use nutrition to put the body in the right state. As many of the triggers for strength or endurance gains are nutritional this means that we can control them pretty well by adapting what and when we eat. The most powerful of these plans involves the ability to switch the body from its endurance adaptation environment to a strength training environment. If we consume carbohydrate to replenish our glycogen stores we have immediately removed one of the biggest inhibitors of our body being able to turn protein into stronger muscle. The next step involves consuming some protein, ideally a high-quality source that is rich in essential amino acids (such as a good supplement). This gives the body a green light to go ahead and start the processes that will result in us getting stronger.

- Finish on the session that matters most. We must accept that unless we train very infrequently there may be a small blunting of the previous training session when we work strength and endurance back-to-back even though this will be minimised by spacing them far apart. The best approach is to finish on the session that is most important to you and not put key sessions close together. Given that you will almost certainly do more endurance than strength work this means putting one of the less important endurance sessions before a key weights session.

- If all else fails, endurance–strength beats strength–endurance. Unless you have the luxury of being a full-time triathlete sometimes life just doesn't allow for perfect planning of training sessions and it becomes necessary to get the sessions in whenever possible. When we reach this point of having to pair two sessions the golden rule is to train endurance first, followed by strength as this has been shown to give the best balance of the two sessions. On the other hand strength followed by endurance has a severely detrimental effect on the strength session.

2.3 The strength argument

It is important to have a good understanding of exactly how strength training may complement endurance performance. Speed and power are not terms that are commonly used in association with endurance sports. Generally we tend to focus on how 'fit' we need to be. However numerous studies have shown that aerobic fitness is actually a very poor predictor of performance. In an Ironman triathlon the VO_2 max of the competitors is generally fairly similar. However the times during each discipline vary enormously. Perhaps the most famous example of this is the Boston marathon performance of seven-times Tour de France winner Lance Armstrong. Despite being one of the greatest cyclists of all time he registered a respectable but unspectacular time of 2 hours 50 minutes. Despite having all of the requisite metabolic fitness for a much faster time, a lack of reactive strength and subsequent running economy appear to have limited performance.

Strength, speed and power

We can argue all day about whether strength, speed and power training can improve endurance performance but ultimately we need to look at the evidence if we really want to take training seriously. Over the past 10 years scientific studies have shown that sprint speeds are a good predictor of 5km times, showing a clear link between pure speed and endurance performance. Similarly we also know that improving our strength qualities will enhance our speed. If this link seems too tenuous there is also a wealth of direct evidence.

A classic study in 1999 by Danish researchers showed gains in endurance running following the introduction of an explosive-strength training programme. What was particularly surprising to many was that rather than simply adding this training to an existing programme it actually replaced some of the previous endurance work. This means that they had proven that not only can strength training aid an endurance training programme but at times it may also be more effective than the traditional work. Since then scores of sports science researchers have found similar findings showing improvements in time trials in both running and cycling.

So if we accept that these types of training will help our performance, the next question is surely, how do they work? The answer lies in the word 'economy'. Almost all of the studies we have talked about have found that cyclists and runners who have carried out strength programmes have improved their cycling and running economy. Very simply this means that they are able to exercise at the same speed at a much lower oxygen cost. This is a far better predictor of performance than the old-fashioned VO_2 max. When you think about it this makes perfect sense. Consider the example of a triathlete who has a top running speed of 16kph. If he runs at 8kph he will be at 50 per cent. If he follows a strengthening programme that improves his top speed to 20kph all of a sudden 8kph is only

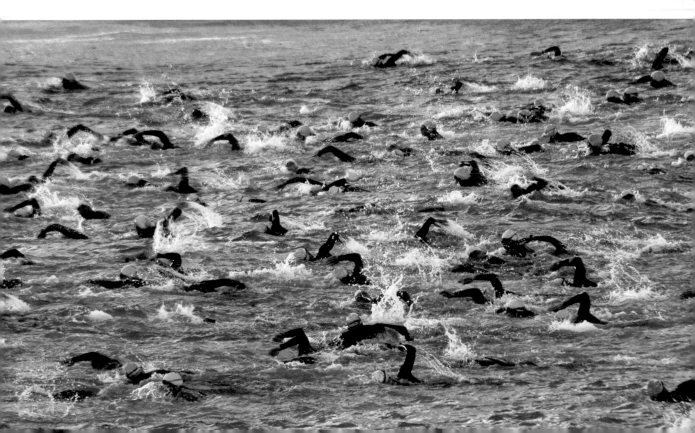

40 per cent of his top speed. Therefore he will need to use less of his fitness capacity even if he doesn't change his aerobic fitness at all. This is a slightly crude example, but it demonstrates the importance of having a 'speed reserve', which enables the athlete to work more efficiently.

You may have noticed that most of the scientific studies discussed are focused on running and cycling. This is not to say that the same benefits are not achievable in swimming. Instead it is probably a reflection of the fact that measuring economy is much more complicated in swimming and researchers tend to favour the easy answer!

As well as improving our speed reserve, our economy can also be improved through improving our mechanical efficiency. Sadly mechanics are often neglected by endurance coaches, particularly when it comes to running. While the enlightened triathlete may well recognise that swimming is a highly technical event, others still continue to work harder than they need to and churn up and down the pool. The situation is often worse in the cycle. Many fail to see the irony that having spent thousands of pounds on precision-engineered bikes their own mechanical efficiency is more like an old post bike than the machine they ride on. Finally we have the worst offender of all – the run. The word 'run' is commonly used to mean a consistent activity. However a short time at any local park will clearly reveal that running techniques are like snow flakes – no two are identical. Sadly the majority are not only unique but also highly inefficient. Mechanics largely go ignored in favour of more minutes on the stopwatch and kilometres on the road.

We can break mechanical efficiency down further into external and internal efficiency. External

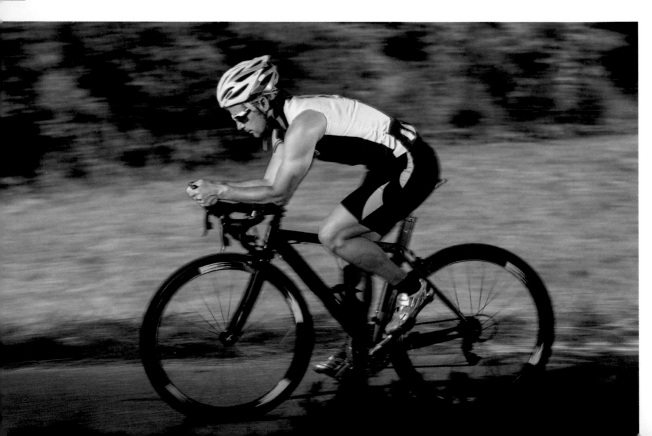

efficiency basically relates to our gross technique and can be assessed by simply watching us perform the disciplines. Typical examples include our ability to hold a streamlined position through the water, having the strength to avoid rolling shoulders on the bike and how well we use reactive strength to make our running look effortless. Internal efficiency is harder to observe but is no less important. We have already learned in chapter 1 than one of the initial adaptations to a strength training programme is greater coordination of muscle groups. In order to move effectively it is just as important for our muscles to 'know' when to relax as it is for them to be able to contract. As we become more skilful at this our movements become more and more effortless. Therefore those who think that endurance sports do not require any skill should think again. A big contributor to this skill is our postural strength and the ability to use our postural muscles correctly and allow the superficial muscles to get on with the job of moving us around the course as quickly as possible.

Despite all of the evidence now available to us, the cynical triathlete will still feel that on any given day their time is better spent running, cycling or swimming than working on their strength or mechanics. What this athlete has failed to realise is that their aerobic training is going to yield increasingly small gains due to the inevitable law of diminishing returns. Going from little or no aerobic training to a moderate amount produces big gains in fitness and performance. However going from moderate to high or from high to very high volumes will produce smaller and smaller improvements. This is when the mechanisms by which strength training improves performance (as discussed in chapter 1) become critical. All of the sports science studies previously discussed have found that strength training programmes have improved performance without any change in aerobic fitness (VO_2 max). This is a crucial piece of information as it proves that strength training allows us to develop an untapped source of performance gain.

2.4 Courage to change

So, now that we have established that a strength programme offers genuine performance gains we must broach the really difficult question: 'What are you going to drop?' This is often the biggest barrier to a successful S&C programme for many triathletes. If an athlete is already training to their full capacity, adding additional sessions in the form of S&C would potentially put them into a state of excessive training stress. This is where the commitment to a strength training programme is truly tested. Of course this may not always be the case as it depends on the current level of training and the athlete's capacity to recover. However for those for whom something has to give the evidence should provide some comfort.

The majority of sports scientists have compared groups whereby one performs an endurance programme and the other does the same endurance programme with one or more sessions replaced by strength sessions. Despite reducing the endurance work, sometimes by up to 20 per cent, the strength groups inevitably make improvements over the endurance-only group. What is even more interesting is that training programmes that have simply added on a strength session on top of normal training generally yield worse results than when a session is removed.

It is clear that the days of a top-quality triathlon training regime simply involving the pool, the bike and the road are now over.

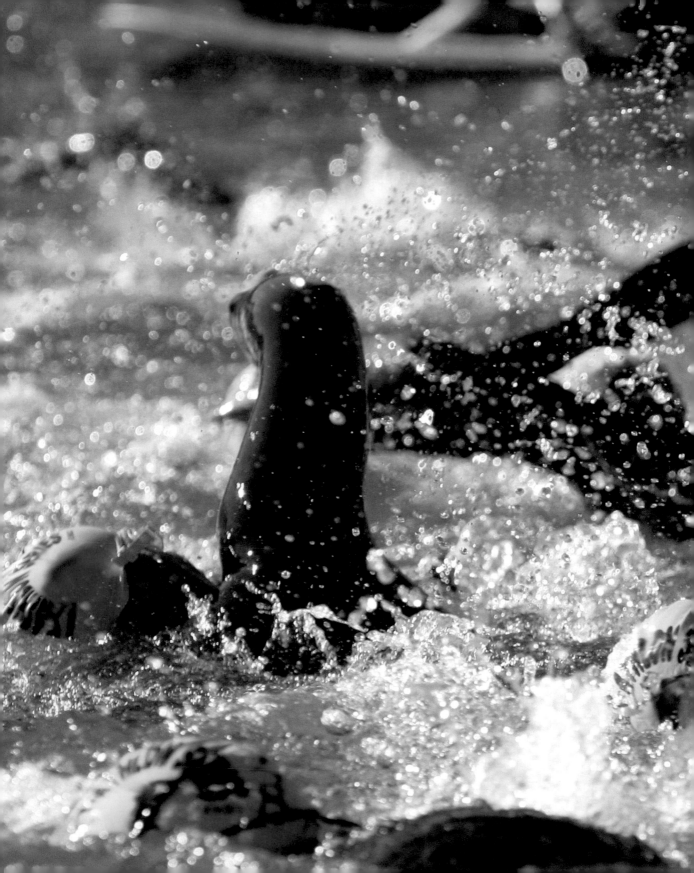

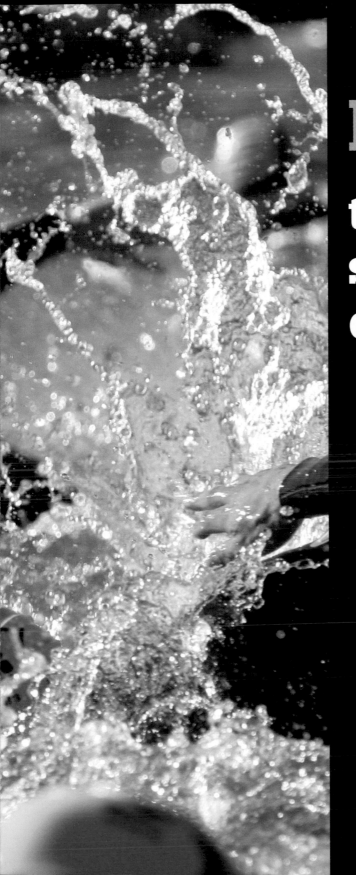

part 2

triathlon strength and conditioning

003
injury prevention

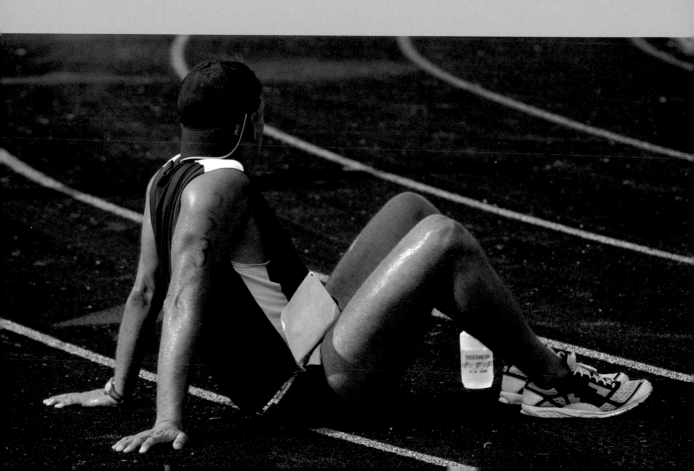

3.1 Introduction

Whether triathlon is a weekend hobby or an Olympic ambition there can be no greater priority for an S&C programme than injury prevention. For the serious athlete this should not be seen as a compromise to performance-enhancing work. Making steady year-on-year progression is by far the best route for any athlete to fulfil their potential. Those who fail to do so are most commonly the victims of injury setbacks, which mean missed or compromised training and crucial years lost to stagnant growth. For the recreational athlete who is less concerned with elite performance and more interested in participation the importance of injury prevention is equally high. For these individuals it is generally the case that injury and an inability to train are ultimately the reasons they reluctantly decide they can no longer take part in the sport they love.

The focus of this chapter is very much on prevention of injury (prehab) rather than rehabilitation. Rehabilitation requires a precise and individualised approach and a proper clinical diagnosis. Athletes who have suffered an injury are urged to seek a good sports physiotherapist as early as possible. The quality of exercise therapy during late-stage rehab does vary dramatically between physiotherapists. Therefore it is important to find someone who not only has a lot of experience of dealing with similar athletes but also a track record of getting athletes back into full fitness effectively. Word of mouth is probably the best way of finding such a person.

3.2 Causes of injury and common problems

Clearly no S&C programme can prevent contact injuries such as bike crashes. Instead we are more concerned with so-called overuse injuries (although perhaps overmisuse may be a better term). There are essentially two reasons for sustaining an overuse injury as a triathlete: dysfunction and poor tissue tolerance. A good S&C regime will address both of these.

Dysfunction is a term that means that our body's mechanics are not optimised. When certain areas of the body become excessively tight or weak we become imbalanced and other areas are stressed as a result. Sometimes the degree of imbalance will be minor and will either cause no issues at all or our bodies will adapt accordingly and so there is no problem. None of us has perfectly balanced bodies, which always move perfectly (even world-class athletes), and so examples of these minor imbalances can be found all over our bodies. When we are able to cope with an imperfect movement it is known as self-optimisation. This is not always the case though, and often an imbalance in the body starts to put sufficient stress on an area that it will ultimately break. For the sedentary individual this is often not a problem as their low level of activity means that the stresses are small and infrequent. However with endurance sports such as triathlon the same actions can be repeated many thousands of times in a single training session. The more we train, the greater the accumulated stress and the greater the risk of injury.

Poor tissue tolerance can apply to muscles as well as tendons, ligaments and even bones. If these tissues are not used to exposure to stress (i.e. training) then they will not recover sufficiently from training and so the athlete goes into the next session with areas of damage. This cycle continues until ultimately an injury occurs. This type of situation is particularly common when someone begins training for the first time or when training is increased at too fast a rate. Ultimately though we will all have a physical ceiling for training, and the more we train the greater the risk of going beyond this point. Of course the physical ceiling will be lowered considerably if we add movement dysfunction, so both of these factors must be dealt with. Increasing tissue tolerance is often the quickest route to dealing with a dysfunction. Changing movement patterns can be a slow process and so improving our ability to cope with them is always a good insurance policy.

Causes of dysfunction

As we have seen movement dysfunction comes about when muscles and connective tissue are too tight, too weak or too long. But how did they get that way in the first place? The answer often lies in the convenience of modern life and the unnatural way in which we treat our bodies for large periods of time. When we are born our bodies are well balanced (from a muscle point of view) and highly mobile. Next time you are with a toddler, watch them squat down to pick something up. Their range of movement would put even the most flexible athlete to shame (*see* figure 3.1).

The problem is that as we grow older we also get lazy. We stop using these fantastic ranges of movement, and as a result we lose them. The exception to this can be seen in some south-east Asian countries, where it is normal to sit in a full squat position; consequently even the average man on the street has fantastic mobility. However in the Western world we are far too fond of the chair. Whether it be at a school desk, in a car, at the office or on the sofa, we spend a phenomenal amount of time sitting down. This leads to a series of adaptations known as lower crossed syndrome (*see* figure 3.2).

The posture shown in figure 3.2 may look worryingly familiar. As you can see, a number of factors combine to make up the condition. Because of large amounts of sitting the hip flexors (illiopsoas) shorten and become tight. This in turn causes the pelvis to rotate forward, lengthening the lower abdominals, which are then inhibited and weak. This rotation of the pelvis also causes the glutes to become less effective, while the hamstrings become tight. The effects are not limited to the lower body either. The familiar slouched position that so many of us are guilty of causes havoc in the upper body. The pectorals start to shorten, drawing the shoulders into a rounded position. This causes the muscles of the upper back to become long and weak. In order to keep balanced the head comes forward which leaves the neck muscles long and tight. It is highly likely that any athlete who has visited a physiotherapist for an overuse injury will have heard at least one of these symptoms already.

Figure 3.1 Baby squat

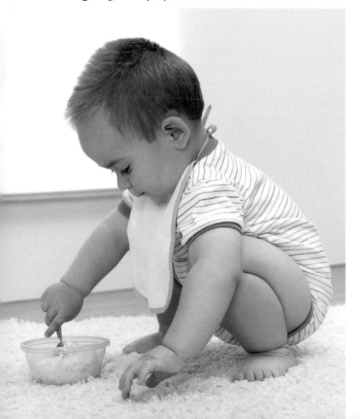

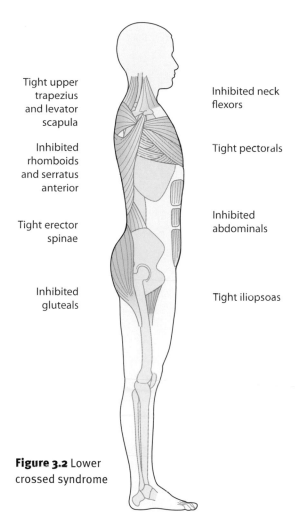

Tight upper
trapezius
and levator
scapula

Inhibited neck
flexors

Inhibited
rhomboids
and serratus
anterior

Tight pectorals

Tight erector
spinae

Inhibited
abdominals

Inhibited
gluteals

Tight iliopsoas

Figure 3.2 Lower
crossed syndrome

that they are kept in good health. When the natural mechanics of the foot are compromised in this way we lose some of the power generated by our hips and thighs. The foot also loses some of its ability to dissipate force, which means it must be taken somewhere else in the body. This can lead to issues around the hips and knees.

Stiff ankles (limited dorsiflexion)
Another common problem of a sedentary lifestyle is stiff ankles. In simple terms this means that the ankle cannot flex the foot towards the shin as much as it needs to. As a result when performing any activity that involves several joints the lack of movement in the ankles must be compensated for elsewhere. Once again this will commonly result in more movements in the knees or lower back. When performing squatting movements the athlete is likely to have an excessive forward lean and the heels will possibly come off the floor.

Knee valgus
This is the term used to describe the movement of the knee falling inward. It most commonly happens when the knee is flexed by a reasonable amount such as walking up stairs or during squatting and lunge exercises. This can cause a lot of problems around the knee. The falling in movement may not appear obvious to the untrained eye during cycling and running, but even minor deviations from the optimal movement can accumulate over many kilometres of training. The dysfunction can arise from several issues, including poor foot and ankle control and unstable hips. The knee itself is rarely the primary cause.

Hip mobility
Mobility of the hips is another movement quality that is most commonly exposed during exercises such as squats and lunges. The importance of hip mobility in the triathlete can easily be overlooked.

This is in no way the only form of dysfunction, but to go through all possible movement issues and their causes is way beyond the scope of this book. However there are a number of very common issues that we can look at.

Common dysfunctions
Flat feet (pes planus)
This is a common condition whereby the arch of the foot 'collapses' as the muscles of the foot have become weak and stretched. As our feet are the only thing that contact either the ground when running or the pedals when cycling it is important

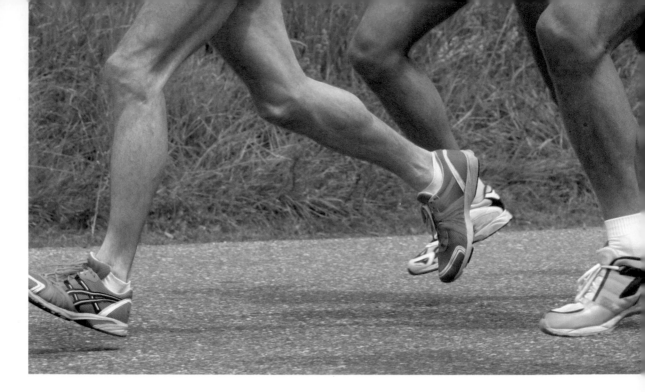

None of the disciplines involve taking our hips through their full range of motion, and so it is commonly assumed that we do not need to work through these ranges. However if a coach understands functional anatomy he will be aware that much of the hip musculature, such as the gluteals, become most active when we are in positions of deep flexion. When we consider some of the common dysfunctions described above the significance of this becomes clear. Therefore it is important that we not only maintain good hip mobility but also train within these ranges.

Pelvic control

As we've already learned, many of our everyday lifestyles lead to a compromise in our pelvic control. The pelvis is an area of the body of primary importance, as almost all movement comes through the pelvis. It has been described as a 'transmission box' with three critical levers coming from it – our two legs and our spine. Relatively small movements in the pelvis will have dramatic effects on all of these levers and

therefore a profound effect on our ability to produce and control force. These small movements in the pelvis are often difficult to identify due to their subtlety, but their effects on other parts of the body are stark. This often results in an assumption that the fault lies in the affected part of the body rather than the pelvic control. Possibly the best example of this comes from the much misunderstood 'core stability' (*see* p. 38). Lack of pelvic control can result in a variety of movements, partly depending on the movement being performed. These include shifting (left or right), tilting (rotating forward or backward), hiking (lifting one side higher than the other) and rotating (left or right in front of the opposite side). To complicate matters further all of these movements will naturally happen to some extent, so we are concerned only when these movements are excessive or uncontrolled.

Thoracic rigidity

Yet another factor of everyday life is thoracic rigidity. However this issue is perhaps unique in

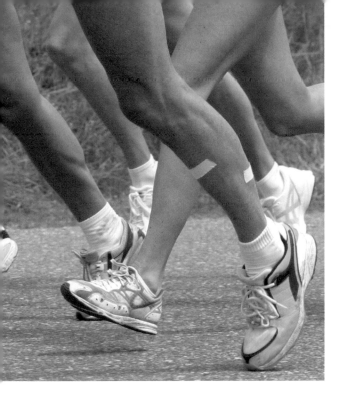

back posture many of us exhibit. The failure to control the scapula properly means that the mechanics of the shoulder joint (where the scapula and the humerus meet) are compromised. This may lead to an issue known as impingement, whereby tendons become 'pinched'.

Internally rotated humerus

Another shoulder condition relating to poor posture is internally rotated humerus. When standing in a relaxed position the palms of the hands should naturally face towards each other. However if the humerus has become internally rotated then the palms will start to face towards the rear. As with scapular winging this may result in a compromise to the smooth flow of the shoulder, and tendons becoming impinged.

that some of our training, in the form of cycling, may actually exacerbate the issue. Our constant sitting and lack of movement can result in the thoracic spine (between the lower back and the neck) becoming very stiff. Consequently we find that we cannot lift the chest or rotate the shoulders to the degree we need, so we try to find the movement from elsewhere. Generally this compensatory range comes from the lower back and the shoulders. This can frequently be seen during swimming, and results in significant stress being placed on the shoulder – the most commonly injured site in the swimmer.

Scapular winging

This describes a condition whereby the scapula (shoulder blade) does not sit as flatly on the rib cage as it should. This can be seen quite clearly when the border of the scapula protrudes out from the back, often when we start to move our arms. The main cause for the condition is an inhibition of the serratus anterior muscle, which once again comes about through adaptations to the rounded

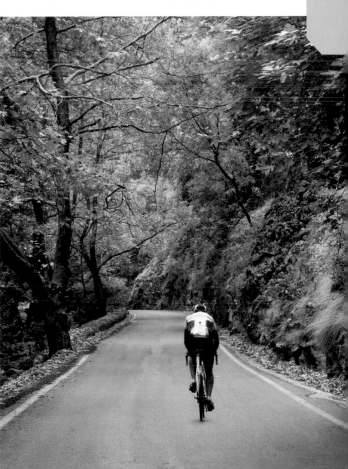

3.3 Identifying risk

So now that we are aware of the importance of injury we need a system to allow us to identify not only how at risk we are but crucially where our vulnerability lies. In order to do this thoroughly we need to assess both movement quality and muscular conditioning. A number of tools are available to make this assessment.

Movement quality

A number of 'movement screens' are now used by coaches to assess the general movement quality of athletes. This process is somewhat controversial, and coaches and physiotherapists often disagree on its use, even though the research evidence is equivocal at the moment. Some researchers suggest that a movement screen can be used to predict injury risk, whereas others feel that the movements are too far removed from sports activity and that the assumptions made are too great. It is certainly true that there are elite athletes who score poorly in these tests who do not get injured and some who score well and are frequently hurt. On the other hand addressing movement issues raised by the tests certainly won't do any harm and may help to reduce mechanical strain. If a dysfunction is identified that relates to an injury

issue then it would certainly be foolhardy not to address it. The specific tests used may vary, but there are general areas that should be reviewed. These include posture, squat pattern, single-leg stability, lumbo-pelvic control, trunk strength and shoulder function. When working with an S&C coach you should expect some form of movement assessment to be part of the initial screening.

Muscular conditioning tests

As well as assessing movement quality it is also important to evaluate conditioning and muscular endurance. This not only gives an indication of tissue tolerance but will also have implications for our ability to maintain good movement patterns under fatigue. This is clearly important as the one thing that can be guaranteed with triathlon is fatigue. The tests described below give a good indication of the conditioning of crucial muscle groups in a movement challenge that is relevant to the task they perform when training. Ideally the tests are performed with a partner or coach, who can time or count repetitions and check for good form. While the tests will involve some degree of fatigue and discomfort, none of them should be performed in the presence of pain. A guide to target scores in the tests is given in table 3.1.

Table 3.1	Guidelines to muscular conditioning tests		
Exercise	**Poor**	**Adequate**	**Excellent**
Prone extension hold	<1 min	90–120 seconds	3 minutes+
Double leg lower	<10	10–20	25+
Calf raise	<10	10–20	25+
Press-ups	<10 (m), <5 (f)	15–20(m), 5–10 (f)	30 (m), 10 (f)
Inverse pulls	<10 (m), <5 (f)	15–20(m), 5–10 (f)	30 (m), 10 (f)

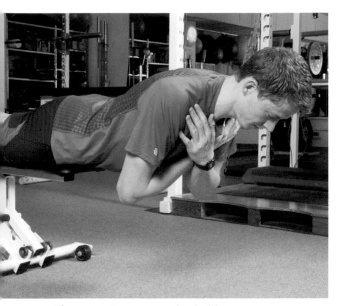

Figure 3.3 Prone extension hold

Prone extension hold

This test gives a good indication of the endurance across the back chain. It is a common area of weakness and can compromise training and racing technique and increase the risk of injury. A bench is needed for this test, as well as a partner to provide resistance. The athlete should lie on the bench face down with the top of the hips just off the bench. The athlete must hold a horizontal position, with arms across the chest, for as long as possible. The body should not be arched excessively beyond parallel; nor should it drop below this position. In order to improve strength of the back chain the athlete should utilise movements such front squats, good mornings and dead lifts (*see* chapter 10).

Double leg lower

This is an excellent test for trunk strength and pelvic control. These areas are required to remain stable while the legs move – precisely the challenge we face during all three disciplines of triathlon.

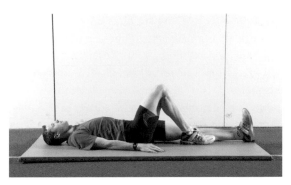

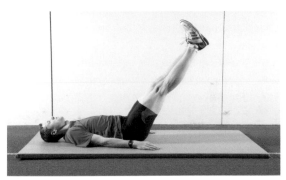

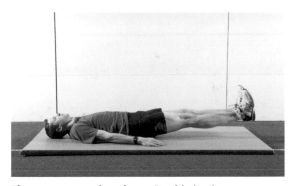

Figures 3.4a, 3.4b and 3.4c Double leg lower

To start the test the athlete must lie on their back and bring the ankle of one leg next to the knee of the other. This leg is then also bent so that the feet are side by side. The legs are then straightened while keeping the thighs at the same angle. The coach will place their hand on the athlete's thigh to give an indication of the start position to return to.

To perform the test the athlete slowly lowers the legs under control to the ground and back to the start position without resting the legs on the floor. The challenge is to perform as many repetitions as possible. The test ends when the athlete cannot perform any more repetitions, experiences pain or cannot maintain a flat lower back and pelvis on the floor. It is also important that the athlete does not feel as if the work is being generated by the back. This also constitutes a fail and is an indication that low-level postural muscles are failing to control forces around the spine.

A poor score in the double leg lower test is best addressed through low-level trunk conditioning work. This can carefully be increased while ensuring that form is excellent and that work feels like it is being generated by the abdominal muscles rather than the back. Exercise progressions include dead bugs, aleknas, plank variations and double leg lowers (*see* chapter 9).

Calf raise
The calf raise is a very simple test to assess the conditioning of the lower leg. The test is also a good indicator of overall muscular conditioning. Test data on elite track and field athletes has shown that conditioning levels throughout the body are well correlated. Therefore a poor score in this test suggests that there may also be a benefit from an all-round conditioning regime.

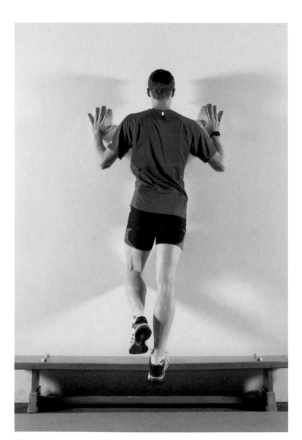 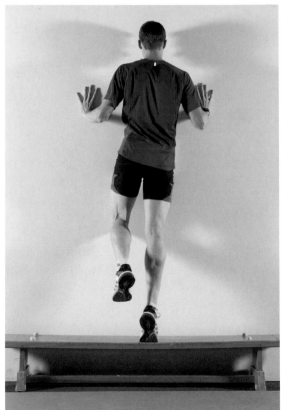

Figures 3.5a and 3.5b Calf raise

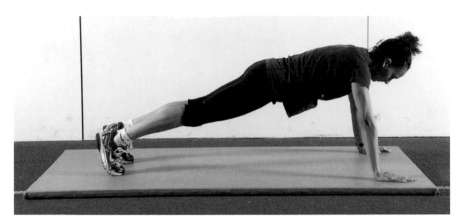

Figure 3.6a
Good-quality press-up

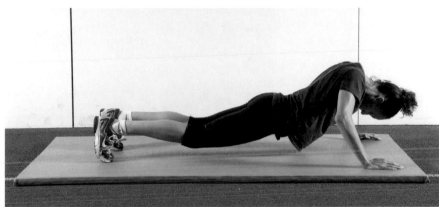

Figure 3.6b
Poor-quality press-up

The athlete stands with the ball of one foot on a step with the opposite foot hanging free. The hands can be placed on a wall for balance, but finder tips should be used to avoid cheating. Starting with the heel dropped to its lowest point the athlete slowly extends the ankle until they are up on their toes before slowly descending back to the start position. The test score is based on the maximum number of repetitions performed to full range. Not only is the absolute score important but also any asymmetries (left–right differences). This should not be greater than 5 per cent. Performing the test to failure often results in significant muscle soreness for the next few days, so it is wise to be selective as to when the test is carried out.

A poor score can be addressed through calf raises themselves (double- or single-legged). It may also be wise to accompany these with other lower leg exercises such as tibialis anterior raises (*see* chapter 9) to ensure a muscle balance.

Press-ups
This very simple and popular exercise can reveal a great deal. It is also much abused and often poorly performed. Essentially it is a test of upper body strength but also requires the strength and endurance of the upper body to be matched by the trunk. The same applies during triathlon.

The press-ups can be performed either from the knees or from the toes depending on strength levels. If fewer than five good full press-ups can be performed then the easier version should be used. All repetitions should be performed under control, at a steady tempo and always to full range. The test reaches a technical fail if the hips start to sag or the chin pokes excessively.

The way in which this test is terminated will dictate the way in which training can be used to improve it. If the athlete simply cannot perform any more reps then the upper body is the limiting factor. Exercises such as press-up variations, pull-ups (*see* chapter 10) and rope climbing are excellent ways of improving relative strength. However if the test ended due to a technical fail then the exercises recommended above for the double leg lower

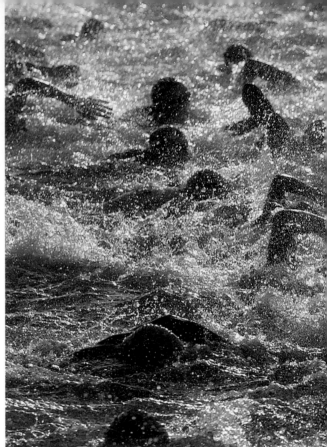

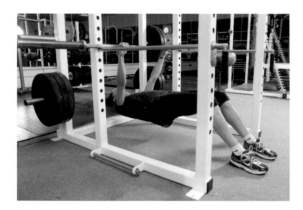

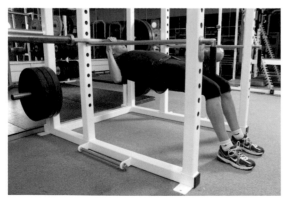

test should be combined with these upper body movements.

Inverse pulls
While the press-up challenge will test pushing strength and the anterior trunk (abs), the inverse pull hold test will assess pulling strength and the lower back. The upper back is commonly a weak area due to the postural issues discussed above.

On a squat rack or Smith machine fix the bar to approximately mid-thigh height. Using an overhand grip the athlete must pull themselves to the bar until the chest bone (sternum) touches the bar. Many will struggle to reach this full range of movement, indicating that the scapular retractors

Figures 3.7a and 3.7b
Inverse pulls

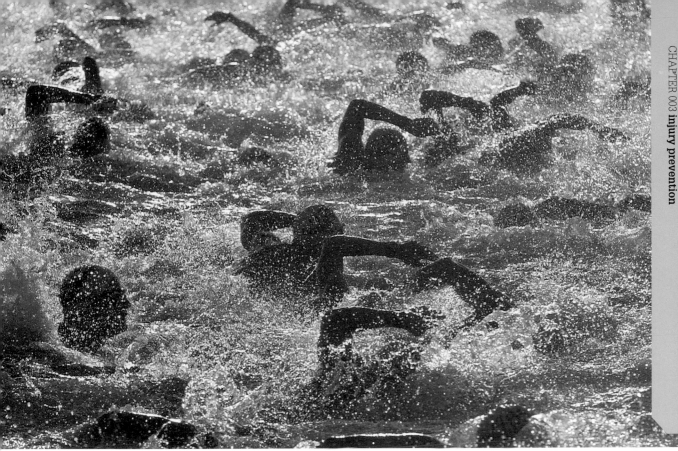

are weak. Often this is compensated for by generating momentum at the bottom of the movement. Therefore the movement should be slow and controlled throughout. Other key technical errors include poking of the chin and arching the back to lift the chest. The tester should record the number of full range repetitions.

Poor performance in the test is most commonly as a result of reduced strength in the upper back at end of range. To address this use exercises that are light enough to allow control at the end of range. Although body weight exercises are generally recommended, these are often too intense to allow the end of range to be effectively targeted in weaker athletes. This can be overcome by offering assistance: for example, by giving light assistance during an inverse pull an athlete can then complete the movement without having to

'cheat' through compensation. Alternatively exercises such as face pulls and Bruce Lees (*see* chapter 9) will precisely target the weakness.

As well as the absolute score, the ratio of push-to-pull strength (i.e. press-ups to inverse pulls) should also be as close as possible to 1:1.

3.4 Prevention routines and case studies

While the individual make-up of each triathlete is unique there are injury-related themes that commonly occur. This section will look at exercise and warm-up routines, which will offer triathletes protection against these issues, through the use of real-life case studies.

CASE STUDY THE ATHLETE WITH WEAK GLUTES

Pauline is a 35-year-old triathlete. She took up the sport after having her second child as a way to get back into shape. She had been a good swimmer in her teens but had always had problems with running. After several months of training Pauline started to experience knee pain and went to see a physiotherapist. She was told that the problem was very common and was a result of her having weak glutes. The physiotherapist gave her a programme of floor-based exercises to target the glutes. While these seemed to hit the right areas when being performed they did little to help the knee pain during running, which continued to deteriorate.

This scenario is extremely commonplace. Pauline is unable to control her knee when running. As her foot strikes the floor the knee drifts inward, placing stress on several ligaments of the knee. It may be that her glutes are weak and will benefit from strengthening; however the gap between their role in floor exercises and that in running is large and must be bridged. Often the problem is a lack of motor control rather than strength *per se*. Therefore Pauline needs exercises that enable her body to practise holding the correct positions in a controlled manner. The example programme below will provide her with suitable control and can also be used prior to running sessions in order to rehearse the movements.

1	Hurdle walk-throughs (*see* p. 180)	3 x 6
2	Lunge walk (*see* p. 133)	3 x 12
3	Diagonal hop-stick (*see* p. 134)	3 x 12
4	Band walks (*see* p. 115)	3 x 10m
5	A-march (*see* p. 178)	3 x 20m
6	Bulgarian squat (*see* p. 162)	3 x 8 x bw*

Note: performed as a circuit

* bw means that no added resistence (i.e. bar or dumbell) is used.

In addition to the above exercises Pauline may also find that her problems are eased if she uses a foam roller to treat trigger points in her ITB (iliotibial band) (*see* chapter 9).

CASE STUDY THE ATHLETE WITH SHOULDER IMPINGEMENT

Chris has been participating in triathlon for five years and has improved his personal best over the Olympic distance each year. At the start of this season he decided the best way to make further gains would be to target the swim, by strengthening his upper body. His brother works in a gym and gave him some popular shoulder exercises to help his power. Chris enjoyed the training but has recently started to experience pain in his shoulder when he lifts his arm above head height.

Most traditional gym shoulder exercises are designed to work the prime movers of the shoulders such as the deltoids and the upper trapezius. They also tend to utilise movements involving pressing weights above the head. The exercise routines are also intended to build mass in the shoulders. These three factors can potentially be a recipe for disaster for the swimmer. If the prime movers become overdeveloped the fine control of the shoulder can be lost and mechanics are negatively affected. While overhead exercises are not bad *per se* they do carry some level of risk. For many this will never be a problem; some will have very low tolerance whereas others will perform the movements happily for years before they start to experience issues. This is largely a result of the shape of the bone around the shoulder joint and therefore the only way to know for sure is an X-ray.

In order to address his problems Chris will need to stop all of his overhead work to allow the shoulder to recover. Depending on the severity this may also include swimming for a period. He can also take a proactive approach and use a well-designed shoulder programme to target the shoulder stabilisers (*see* below). He may also benefit from soft-tissue treatment around the shoulder from a sports masseur.

1   YTML (*see* p. 147)   3 x 8
2   Swimmers (*see* p. 148)   3 x 12
3   Press-ups (*see* p. 166)   3 x 10
4   Scap press-ups (*see* p. 149) 3 x 20

CASE STUDY THE ATHLETE WITH POOR FLEXIBILITY

Tom was a fairly typical recreational athlete when it came to flexibility. He would always stretch for around five minutes before training and sometimes afterwards too. However despite this he always felt like he should probably do more. Tom wasn't sure exactly how flexible he needed to be but generally considered himself to be too stiff. Occasionally he would make a concerted effort to improve his flexibility and stretch a little longer. After several weeks though he saw no difference and gradually went back to his old routine.

There are few of us who do not wish that we were slightly more flexible. However the timing and type of stretching we do is critical if we are to make improvements. We can discuss this in terms of three categories: pre-training stretches, post-training stretches and developmental stretching.

Pre-training stretching has become a topic of much debate in recent years. Not so long ago every coaching course would begin with basic instruction on the importance of carrying out static stretches during the warm-up. These are the traditional type of stretches involving holding a muscle in a stretched position. However there is now a growing body of evidence suggesting that this may not only be unnecessary but could also actually increase the risk of injury and impair performance! The theory behind this is that by stretching the muscles for extended periods the mechanical sensors in the muscle become 'confused'. In simple terms the body loses some of its awareness of the exact positions of joints and so control is reduced and the athlete becomes more vulnerable. The capacity for reactive strength may also be reduced as the stretching may temporarily reduce the elastic qualities of the muscle and tendons. In reality the case against static stretching may have been overstated. It is now clear that athletes certainly don't need to perform static stretches before a session. However many athletes will feel more comfortable, partly through habit, if they have gone through a couple of their favourites. A more in-vogue approach is to warm up using dynamic stretches. These involve moving through ranges of movement in a controlled way without holding the position (*see* below). These have the advantage of working many of the stabilising muscles and may help to 'activate' many muscle groups that become underactive during long periods of sitting through the day. In general the higher the intensity of the session the more likely a dynamic warm-up is to be appropriate. Whatever the preference, stretching prior to the session should only ever be considered preparatory work – i.e., the stretches are aimed at readying the athlete for the session rather than achieving long-term improvements in flexibility.

Post-training stretches can be used to improve long-term flexibility but are also important for recovery and restoring natural length to muscles. During this time static stretches are entirely appropriate. The biggest limitation to developing flexibility here is likely to be fatigue.

Stretching sessions are often cut short or abandoned altogether because of a desire to shower, eat or just collapse!

A developmental stretching session can be performed as a distinct session in its own right. This will ensure that sufficient time and energy are available to focus properly on the task. As well as traditional stretches many triathletes are now including elements of yoga in their flexibility routines. This is not only a very effective method but can also be an efficient way of training, because postural strength may also be developed simultaneously. Attending a well-instructed yoga class is the easiest way of introducing yoga to a programme. Time often makes this impractical though as training for three disciplines on top of normal life is generally enough to keep most of us busy. By using a few selected yoga poses it is still possible to make good progress.

The programme below gives a dynamic warm-up routine, which Chris may find benefits his high-intensity sessions, as well as a developmental stretch routine, which combines yoga and traditional stretches. This can be used post-workout or can be extended to form a session in itself.

Sample dynamic warm-up flexibility routine:

1 Skips (*see* p. 179)   2 x 30m

2 Hamstring march (*see* p. 144)   2 x 15m

3 Lunge walk (*see* p. 133)   2 x 10m

4 Various crawls (*see* p. 135)   2 x 10m

Sample developmental stretches and yoga:

1 Downward dog (*see* p. 136)

2 Sun Salutation (*see* p. 137)

3 Walking glute stretch (*see* p. 145)

4 Hip flexor stretch (*see* p. 143)

5 Basic hamstring stretch (*see* p. 144)

6 Thoracic extension mobiliser (*see* p. 138)

Note: hold each of these stretches for 1–2 minutes and repeat up to three times. Also seek expert instruction on yoga poses.

CASE STUDY THE ATHLETE WITH A WEAK CORE

Manjit had been training for 3–4 years and had entered a number of duathlons and sprint triathlons. Her training had become a bit monotonous and she had never been a fan of winter training so her brother bought her a session with a personal trainer for Christmas. The trainer had told her that her aerobic fitness seemed pretty good but she needed to be more flexible and improve her core stability. She went away and bought herself a physio ball, which had been recommended, and started doing crunches on it and practised balancing. Manjit's performances in all three disciplines stayed pretty static and she wasn't entirely sure how she should feel the benefit.

Situations such as Manjit's are far from rare. Core stability is a term that became popular about 10 years ago and has caused much confusion and debate ever since. This has resulted in some of the most heinous myths in gym culture.

Myth #1: The term 'core' is generally used as a substitute for abdomen. In fact claiming to be doing some core work is often just an excuse for doing some six-pack training! A better definition would be to include the pelvis and the trunk, although it could be argued that the pelvis alone is really the core. As discussed above, pelvic control has a profound effect on what will happen at the trunk, so a stable pelvis equals a stable core.

Myth #2: The second great myth regards a muscle called the transverse abdominus. Until a few years ago many people believed that this muscle must be voluntarily activated before performing sports movements. This resulted in athletes trying to 'switch on' before each exercise in the gym. Although the muscle is important this theory has now been discredited as in reality a number of muscles around the trunk act together to provide stability.

Myth #3: The best way to develop core stability is by sitting on a big ball or by performing exercises on a mat. With the emergence of the idea of core stability came the inevitable commercial drive behind it in the shape of the physio ball. With this also came a range of crazy exercises, which had more to do with the circus than sports performance.

In reality core stability requires the muscles of the pelvis, hips and trunk to be strong, but the athlete must also have excellent motor control of these body parts. The traditional trunk exercises, which many now describe as core stability, have their place in terms of simply making the relevant muscles stronger. This can be used to create what has been described as 'superstiffness'. This type of stability is ideal for activities such as performing heavyweight lifting, when the core must be kept as rigid as possible so the spine is in a healthy position. However many athletes can develop great levels of strength and conditioning in these types of exercise but still look clunky and mechanical when swimming, be unstable when cycling and slump during running. Conversely athletes who look sleek, efficient and controlled in these events fail to excel in conditioning exercises, because stability is movement specific! Naturally the muscles involved must possess an adequate level of strength and capacity. However beyond these adequate levels there is little or nothing to be gained. Those who like to grind out 1,000 sit-ups should take note!

Unlike the superstiffness required when weightlifting, stability in triathlon requires a concept known as 'flow'. An athlete who has flow looks strong and stable yet relaxed and smoothed. Flow enables the athlete to perform perfect technique effortlessly rather than mechanically and under strain. This comes about when the deep postural muscles are performing correctly. These muscles are naturally designed to hold posture for long periods, thus allowing the prime movers to get on with the job of getting us round the course as quickly as possible. The design and natural function of these muscles also give us a clue as to how best to train them. Unlike the postural muscles the prime movers are not effective at maintaining a low level of contraction for a long time. Therefore if we perform low-intensity work for moderate durations (15–20 minutes) one of two things will happen. If we rely on the prime movers they will quickly fatigue and our technique will break down. However if we maintain form for this duration the postural muscles will be targeted and become trained in these movements. Provided that the movements are appropriate to the activity then flow will start to develop. Therefore technical drills with a focus on posture will provide the most natural and specific form of core training.

So, in summary, to develop true core stability for triathlon an athlete requires a threshold level of strength and endurance through the trunk and hips and to develop appropriate motor patterns to enable them to achieve flow in performance. The best way to do these is through a combination of simple but perfectly performed isolation exercises and carefully selected and well-taught drills. In order to be most effective in improving motor control an athlete needs to have an insight into where the flaws in their technique lie (and the underlying physical causes).

CASE STUDY THE ATHLETE WITH BAD FEET AND ANKLES

Clare was a 28-year-old professional triathlete competing at a high level. Over the past two years she has suffered from various low-level knee and ankle problems and also has painful feet if she stands up for too long. Her coach arranged for her to have a biomechanical assessment. This revealed that she had excessive pronation when running, so she has been advised to start using orthotics. Even though this advice seemed to make sense Clare was unsure how to proceed as she knew several triathletes who had had bad experiences with orthotics.

The use of orthotics is a contentious issue, with much depending on the expertise of the podiatrist and the athlete's own personal circumstances. While they are often a powerful aid, a better more permanent solution may be to improve the health of the foot and ankle control. The foot is actually a cleverly engineered structure, which is able to reduce the impact forces of running as well as storing and reusing energy. In order to maintain this structure the feet must be kept in good health and the intrinsic muscles must be kept conditioned. Possibly the simplest form of exercise for the feet is to perform some bare-foot work. The support provided by most modern shoes (cycling, running and regular shoes) can result in the feet becoming 'lazy'. Try performing simple exercises such as lunges in bare feet. You will most likely see the feet twitching and flicking as the intrinsic muscles wake up and start to seek proprioceptive feedback to support the foot. This challenge can be further increased by performing work in sand (either the beach or a long-jump pit is ideal). This generalised work also carries the benefit of conditioning the hips and trunk and is therefore very efficient.

For those with specific foot issues a more specific element of foot conditioning may be appropriate. This may include isolated exercises such as towel scrunches and towel toe work (*see* below). Even for those without issues a small amount of foot conditioning work performed as part of a general conditioning programme is a wise investment. Problems further up the body, such as those with the knees and hips, can often be helped or alleviated by optimising mechanics at the foot and ankle.

Sample foot and ankle conditioning routine:

1 Bare-foot lunging (*see* p. 133)

2 Ankle rolls (*see* p. 146)

3 Hop-stick (*see* p. 134)

4 Towel scrunches (*see* p. 142)

5 Tib ant raises (*see* p. 120)

6 Calf raises (both kinds) (*see* pp. 116 and 117)

CASE STUDY THE ATHLETE WITH NOTHING WRONG WHO WANTS TO KEEP IT THAT WAY!

The best conditioning programme is one that prevents an injury, which you never knew you would have had. Therefore the wise athlete will engage in a general prehabilitation routine to ensure that troubles are always kept at arm's length. This can seem daunting. There are so many potential injuries that surely protecting against them all would leave no time for regular training. However the good news is that many of the most common issues are interlinked, so by using compound exercises that target multiple tissues a highly effective and efficient regime can be designed.

A sample general prehab routine:

1   Single-leg PNF pulls (*see* p. 150) – targets single-leg stability, trunk strength and the rotator cuff

2   Press-up to plank (*see* p. 166) – for trunk strength and serratus anterior for shoulder

3   Multi-directional lunge bare footed (*see* p. 133) – for hip conditioning, hip mobility, single-leg stability, foot and ankle conditioning, core stability/flow

4   Superman (*see* p. 126) – for flow through trunk and shoulders

5   Box squats (*see* p. 159) – for hips and trunk conditioning

6   Bruce Lees (*see* p. 152) – excellent isolated shoulder conditioning

7   Sun salutation routine (*see* p. 137) – for all-round mobility and postural strength

004
the swim

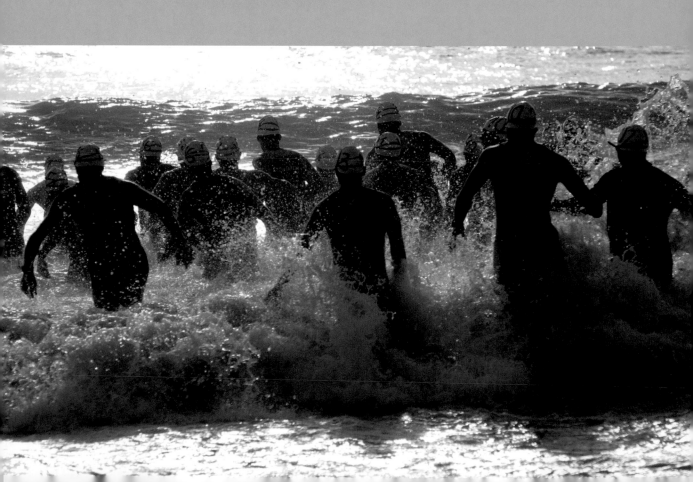

4.1 Introduction

Of the three disciplines that make up triathlon the use of S&C to improve swim performance is perhaps the most controversial. Swimming is clearly a highly technical sport, and a failure to acknowledge this is a common mistake in many novice triathletes. Far too often it is treated like the bike and the run, and athletes simply get in the pool and work hard in the hope that times will come down. In the absence of good technique this is a very flawed and frustrating process. Having said that, there is something of a trend towards 'throwing the baby out with the bath water'. Many popular texts place such a strong emphasis on technical development that physical qualities are completely ignored. A quick glance along the poolside of any swim meet will tell you that this too is unwise.

To add to the confusion there is still much debate around the merits of so-called 'land training'. Because of the highly technical nature of the discipline the transfer of training from the gym to the pool is not as simplistic as it may be with cycling for example. As a result many coaches and swimmers have experimented with S&C or land training over the years in a crude fashion and not surprisingly had poor results. Much of what is currently done is performed more in hope than full confidence that it will work. It is clear then that if we are to have genuine impact on the first of our three disciplines we need to have a clear and precise understanding of exactly what we hope to achieve and the best methods of going about it.

4.2 The technical basis of S&C for swimming

As seen already, much debate exists among swim coaches regarding fitness versus technique. A very simple summary of the challenge faced in swimming comes from a group of researchers who

performed a biomechanical analysis of the front crawl: 'The success of a swimmer is determined by the ability to generate propulsive force, while reducing the resistance to forward motion.' This may seem relatively obvious, but essentially it tells us that both are important rather than there being a single answer.

This simple philosophy indicates two clear pathways to direct our S&C towards improving swim performance: work that helps improve our technique; and work that helps produce more power in the water. It is worth noting that, as with all the disciplines, the reduction of injury risk represents a third category of work that may improve performance. This is discussed in chapter 3. It should be emphasised though that the shoulders really weren't designed to provide locomotion. We have a great range of movement in the shoulder to enable us to reach for things in all directions, but the joint is fundamentally unstable. The higher the volume of swimming performed, the greater the risk to the shoulder. If you are prone to shoulder problems and swim regularly in the pool then this should take priority over the other two elements of training.

The physical demands of good technique

So let us begin with a look at how S&C can have a positive impact on technique. Coordination, experience and the quality of coaching are clearly very important factors in determining a swimmer's technical prowess. It is a mistake to assume that these are the only factors. As with many sporting tasks, good technique is a product of the athlete's motor learning and their physical ability to produce the correct movement patterns. It is with the latter that S&C can have a big impact.

Smooth and effective swimming requires excellent segmental control. This refers to the swimmer's ability to dissociate one body part from another and move only the desired area rather than make clumsy movements involving many areas. This feature distinguishes elite from non-elite swimmers. Those performing at a high level are able to roll from the shoulder while maintaining stable hips, whereas poor swimmers tend to produce the roll from the hips. To perform the movement correctly requires fine motor control around the trunk. If the swimmer has good postural control from the deep core muscles the chances of maintaining segmental control, and therefore technique, during long swims will be much greater. Those who are fearful of spending time on developing this and prefer to churn out length after length will never achieve their full potential as they are simply further enforcing this inefficient pattern.

Segmental control is not the only factor that affects the quality of body roll. In order to produce the desired movement through the shoulders the swimmer must have sufficient thoracic mobility. This term describes the amount of movement possible in the thoracic spine (chest and upper back). The vertebrae in this portion of the spine are well suited to movement and should come second only to the neck in terms of their range of movement. However due to the movement dysfunction caused by daily life (including cycling) it is common that this movement is restricted. A lack of rotation here will mean that a swimmer has to produce the movement from elsewhere – generally at the hips.

If segmental control describes the fine control of the trunk, then trunk strength itself must also be mentioned. This is more to do with preventing than generating movement. The abdominals play a key role in transferring the force generated by the arms and legs effectively. Failure to do so will have a doubly negative effect – not only does the body suffer 'energy leaks' where force is dissipated though unwanted movement, but further drag is also created where the swimmer loses control of the trunk. If trunk strength is poor then the only alternative the swimmer has available is to reduce the power they produce to a level that can be controlled.

This leads us nicely on to shoulder mobility. A restriction in shoulder mobility is terminal to good swimming technique. If a triathlete is unable to hold the arm above the head in line with the body and also bring a recovery arm behind the head then the technical model will always be flawed. Even if these positions can be achieved at a push it is highly likely that technique will not be smooth and the swimmer will be working far harder than is necessary to achieve the right shapes. If the shoulder simply cannot reach this position then

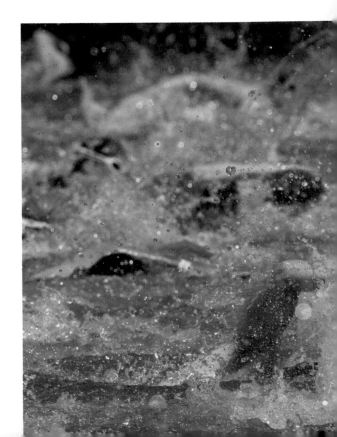

the swimmer is forced to arch the back (thoracic extension) in order to lift the hand high enough. This will immediately increase drag, so technique is compromised.

Complex analysis of swimming mechanics has also revealed that those who use unilateral breathing may start to develop physical asymmetries the longer they continue training. This in turn has also been shown to reduce technical efficiency. The obvious answer to this is to move to a bilateral breathing pattern. However if this is not an appealing or practical thought then the gym is an ideal environment to identify and address any muscular imbalances.

Studies have demonstrated that a 10 per cent improvement in propulsion efficiency versus the same degree of gain in aerobic or anaerobic fitness has a much greater impact on performance. Of course the potential for improvement in each area will influence this. A highly unfit individual with great technique clearly needs to do more work. It seems unlikely that this picture would fit with most triathletes though. An example of this can be seen in the fact that propulsion efficiency has been found to be around 61 per cent in elite swimmers versus just 44 per cent in triathletes.

Before seeking to address any of these issues it is prudent to seek the advice of a competent swim coach, who can provide invaluable insight into the direction and significance of technical deficiency. There is thus much more to good technique than simply knowing what to do and practising it.

The potential to improve propulsion

It is very clear that just because an athlete gets strong in the gym does not automatically mean they will be quicker through the water. Some

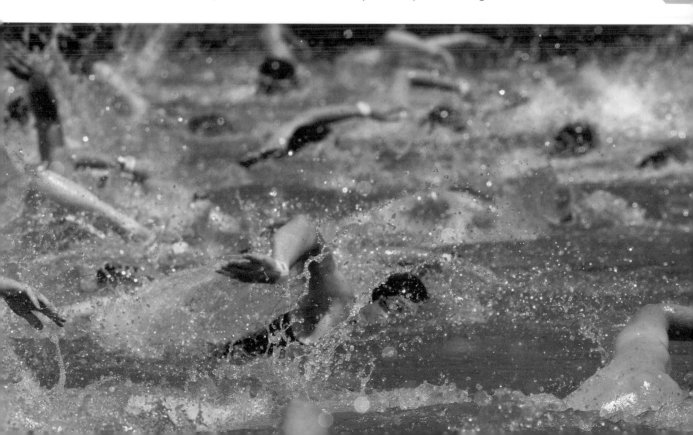

studies have sought to achieve this and found that even with strength gains of 25 per cent the athlete was no quicker in the pool! Therefore to make strength training for swim performance work the athlete needs a good understanding of both strength training methods and swimming. Too often programmes are prescribed by those who have one but not the other. Swimmers who achieved such big gains in strength without getting any quicker may also have found that following a transition period of training they learn to use this new-found strength effectively and speed gains would appear.

Perhaps it makes sense to look at exactly what happens to muscle fibres during swim training. As we start to train, the shortening speed of our slow-twitch muscle fibres increases whereas that of our fast-twitch fibres become slower. This means that our potential for speed and power is reduced. During the taper this process is reversed to some extent. While the slow-twitch fibres generally remain unchanged the fast-twitch fibres show an increased capacity to produce force and shorten more quickly and as a result produce more power. This typically results in an increase in power production of around 10 per cent with performance gains of 4–7 per cent. (The amount of performance gain is related to the level of swimmer and is likely to be linked to their technical ability to utilise the newly gained power.) We therefore know that part of the reason for enhanced performance following a taper is due to greater power production in fast-twitch fibres. This is very important as it means that there is a good theoretical basis for making further performance gains by targeting the power potential of fast-twitch fibres.

A cynic would be quick to point out that while a theoretical basis is great it is certainly not the same as evidence in the real world. Thankfully

there is also good evidence to show that strength gains can in fact be translated to the pool when done effectively. Gains in strength of the elbow extensors and flexors, along with speed in the pool, have been achieved through a variety of resistance training programmes. These include resisted swimming and gym-based exercise. This is important as it means that both modes may be used most effectively in a periodised programme for maximum effect (*see* below). As well as the muscles that produce force at the elbow, the latissimus dorsi is also a muscle of particular interest. This is responsible for a very large component of the pulling force generated by the upper body. It is not surprising then that swimmers who took part in electrical stimulation training of this muscle improved both strength and swim speed. Finally the peak power generated by the arms and legs, even in non-swimming tasks, has been shown to correlate very highly with freestyle swim performance.

Having established not only that strength gains can improve performance but also the muscular mechanisms behind it, surely there can be no argument against it? However some would still question the need to go into the gym and would prefer to do strength work in the pool. While we have already seen that some gains can be made in this way they are still missing out on some of the potential advantages of land-based training. The speed with which the arms move through the water greatly restricts the swimmer's ability to generate high forces. Typically the time in the water allows only 0.3–0.4 seconds to generate force, whereas it takes around double this time to produce maximum force. This has two major implications for training. Firstly by using resistance exercises which allow more time to develop force a greater level of mechanical stress can be placed on the muscles; this is one of the most important

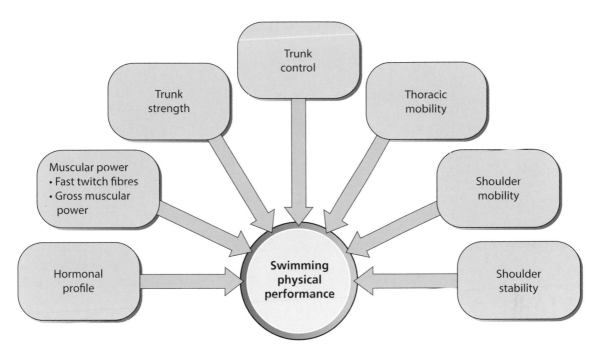

Figure 4.1 Strength factors contributing to swim performance

factors in developing force and power. Secondly, given that the swimmer does not have time to produce maximal force in the water, the rate at which they develop it (rate of force development) becomes a key physical attribute. This can be enhanced through explosive gym-based exercises.

The final barrier to introducing propulsion-enhancing work comes from how it is incorporated into a triathlete's busy schedule. Simply adding sessions to the existing programme is likely to lead to burn out. On the other hand how do we know that gains made in the gym might not have been surpassed by staying in the pool? Thankfully several studies have shown that when the volume of long slow work is reduced and replaced with explosive training there is no negative impact on endurance. There may actually be significant additional benefits to reducing this high-volume work in favour of S&C. High volumes of training

are associated with high levels of cortisol (a hormone that reflects the level of physical stress an individual is under). On the other hand land training has been shown to increase testosterone and potentially reduce cortisol. The testosterone:cortisol ratio is an important marker of the body's capacity to train and perform, so potentially the swimmer will be in better shape to make gains in all other forms of training too!

The potential sources of performance enhancement through strength and conditioning are illustrated in figure 4.1.

4.3 The practical application of S&C to swimming
Now that we have established exactly how physical development on land can impact on swim performance we can start to examine practical

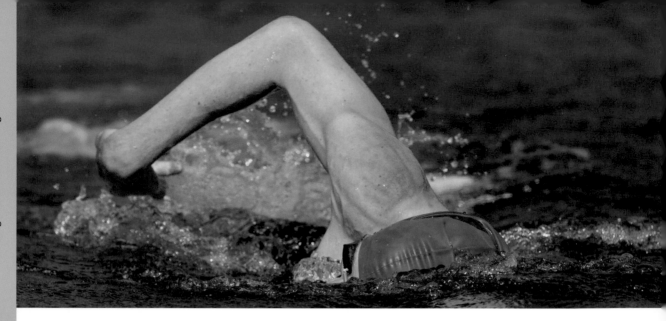

methods of achieving the qualities previously discussed.

Physical development to improve technique

Segmental control

The key to developing segmental control lies in the fact that it is essentially a matter of motor control rather than gross strength. This means that we need to focus on perfection of technique; we do not need to work hard or move large weights. Motor control is also very specific, and so it is also important to train using movements that mimic the sports challenge.

When developing the ability to roll the shoulders to breath efficiently there are a series of rolling exercises that are not only great for developing control but are also useful tests of current levels (see chapter 9). The first challenge is to master the rolling movement (in both directions) in the controlled setting of a mat. Until this can be controlled then attempting to do the same in the pool is highly unlikely to lead to smooth technique. Once good control has been achieved on the floor then rolling swim drills can be incorporated. For some swimmers this will mean

that the floor work can be dispensed with. However others have a lower ability to 'hold on to' training adaptations, and it may be necessary to keep a smaller amount of floor rolling in the programme to avoid regressing.

The woodchop is another movement that is excellent for developing segmental control. This requires much more strength than the rolling exercises. While strength *per se* is not required to attain control the strenuous nature of the exercise helps to reinforce the movement pattern and accelerate learning. However caution must be taken to ensure that excellent technique is not compromised just to muscle the repetitions out. The Swiss ball Russian twist can also be used to the same effect. Again the emphasis is on keeping the hips still while the shoulders roll.

As well as developing rotational control the swimmer also requires lumbo-pelvic dissociation. This will affect the ability to kick hard with the legs without arching the back. The ideal exercise for practising this is the Superman. As with the rolling exercises this can ultimately be progressed to the pool for greater specificity. Here float kicking exercises can be used to great effect. In order to get the most benefit the swimmer should concentrate on maximising the kick while controlling the trunk position (i.e., not allowing the back to arch).

Thoracic and shoulder mobility

The exercises used to develop thoracic and shoulder mobility are relatively quick and simple. This means that for efficiency of training they can be incorporated into other sessions such as during the warm-up. This is particularly effective as part of a swim session warm-up as the short-term increases in mobility will also aid technique within the session.

Try using the following exercises at whatever time of the week is most convenient. Three times per week is probably the minimum requirement to develop greater long-term mobility.

Thoracic exercises

1 Indian sitting with side flexions   3 x 6
   (*see* p. 139)

2 Indian sitting with rotations   3 x 6
   (*see* p. 139)

3 Scorpions (*see* p. 140)   3 x 8

4 Stick/band dislocations (*see* p. 153)   2 x 8

Trunk strength

The challenge for the trunk during swimming is to transfer forces effectively by remaining stable while the arms and legs move. Therefore it is sensible to select exercises that reflect this. There are probably more exercises for this part of the body than any other. Most of these tend to be variations on the sit-up or crunch, and programmes generally focus on the abdominals rather than the lower back. In order to maximise trunk stability a balance of strength in both the front and the back of the body is required. I have seen swimmers who have ignored this principle and were able to perform 1,000 sit-ups but fewer than 10 dorsal raises! Suffice to say this does not reflect smart training. It is worth mentioning that whole body barbell exercises such as squats are often a way in which the back can become strong without additional exercises. However if this type of work is not included in the wider programme then a front and back approach to trunk training is necessary.

The sample routine in table 4.1 is designed on three levels. The routine covers all aspects of the trunk in a manner that is relevant to swimming. The three levels provide progression as trunk strength is developed. The best approach is to begin at the lowest level and progress, rather than

Table 4.1	Some swimming trunk-strength progressions	
Level 1	**Level 2**	**Level 3**
Dead bugs	Aleknas	Weighted aleknas
Body weight squat	Prone extension holds	Prone Superman holds
Modified plank	Front plank	3-point plank
Side plank	Moving side plank	Side plank with leg lifts

attempting to tolerate the higher levels immediately as this may lead to poor technique.

Dealing with asymmetry
Attempting to address an asymmetry is more about how an exercise is performed than the exercise itself. Naturally exercises that address the unbalanced movement must be selected. In many ways these will identify themselves when training for strength and power. The key is to use unilateral exercises rather than bilateral versions. An example of this would be using dumb-bells instead of barbells during upper body exercises. Many commercial gyms now have cable machines with independent handles, which also allow unilateral pulling movements. Even without obvious asymmetries these are always good options for best transfer to performance, as the front crawl swim stroke is a unilateral action.

Physical development to improve propulsion power

Having dealt with the physical issues that relate to improving technique and reducing drag the topic of increasing propulsion is relatively simple – or so it would seem. In order to improve muscular power in a way that will impact on swim performance we need to pay careful attention to exercise selection, movement speed, volumes of work, loadings, etc. What's more, for an athlete to reach their full potential for power production requires careful planning and manipulation of these variables. Making early gains is relatively easy, but these will

soon plateau if the programme isn't progressed and adapted appropriately.

There is a logical sequence of progressions that a programme should follow (*see* figure 4.2). This is also discussed in much greater detail in chapter 7.

The way in which these stages are progressed can be done in two ways. The experienced trainer can go through the various stages during the course of the season. Under this system the special strength work would coincide with the priority races of the season. However for the novice athlete it is recommended that a good base level of general strength is attained before moving on to specific and special strength training methods, regardless of the stage of the season. Without this foundation the benefits of the more advanced stages will be compromised.

General strength and body control
A classic mistake when looking to develop power is to jump straight into explosive exercises performed at speed. These are highly effective but only at the correct time. Power is a combination of force and velocity, or strength and speed in everyday language. Without previous strength training a triathlete's ability to produce maximal force will not be developed. This means that a very low ceiling is placed on their capacity for power production. On the other hand increasing basic strength is likely to have a positive impact on power production as well as acting as a building block for the later stages of training.

Gaining good body control is also an important building block for the latter stages of training. If control is poor then not only will more advanced techniques put the athlete at risk of injury but the exercises will also be less effective. An athlete can become more powerful simply through better mechanics as a result of gaining body control

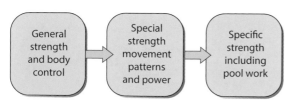

Figure 4.2 Progression of swim strength development

Table 4.2	Some general strength exercises		
Area	**Novice**	**Intermediate**	**Advanced**
Press	Partial press-ups	Press-ups	Deep press-ups
Pull	Bent knee inverse pulls	Inverse pulls	Pull-ups
Legs	Body weight squats	Single-leg squats	Weighted single-leg squats

without actually gaining any strength at all. So how do we develop general strength and body control? The key is to begin with exercises that use body weight as resistance rather than barbells, dumbbells and certainly not machines. As seen earlier, S&C is about training movements rather than muscles. It is important to develop pulling and pushing strength as well as leg strength. During this phase of training it is important to develop the ability to perform these key movements well, and then the ability to do them repeatedly.

The humble press-up is one of the most valuable exercises at our disposal. It also offers a variety of options to increase or decrease the intensity as well as shift the emphasis of the exercise. Pressing movements will not only work the elbow extensors (triceps) but also the chest and shoulders, all of which contribute to propulsion power. The need to maintain good technique also places a great challenge on the trunk. This means that the exercise achieves a number of goals while also developing strength in a manner that has natural carry over to sports performance.

Pulling exercises are slightly more complicated as they tend to be somewhat harder. While almost everyone can perform some variation of a press-up, exercises such as pull-ups are too challenging for many. This issue must be overcome, because

pulling movements arguably represent the single most important component of power production for swimming propulsion. We have already seen that strengthening the latissimus dorsi (lats) can have a beneficial effect on swim performance. This is one of the key pulling muscles, particularly in vertical pulls such as chin-ups. Additionally pulling exercises will also develop strength in the elbow flexors (biceps) and, if performed correctly, improve the strength of the scapular retractors. This can help to address the common movement dysfunction of protracted shoulders and internally rotated humerus (*see* chapter 3). If full pull-ups prove too challenging then a number of variations can be used to regress the exercise. The use of assistance bands can help to off-load body weight to make pull-ups easier. Cable stack machines can also be used to train vertical pulls. However these often result in the athlete flexing the trunk, so the training of this area is somewhat compromised. A horizontal pull such as the inverse pull (*see* chapter 10) will also reduce the amount of body weight that is being lifted, although the contribution of the lats is reduced.

Leg strengthening exercises may possibly be most effective during general strengthening if viewed as 'whole body' exercises. The isolated strengthening of the legs may be of relatively small benefit as the legs remain straight during the freestyle swim.

However exercises such as squats and single-leg squats will develop trunk and whole body control. The debate around the value of this type of work however may be somewhat academic with regard to the triathlete. Even if one is not convinced of the value of leg strength to the swim it is highly likely that this type of work will feature in the overall S&C programme to enhance cycle and run performance.

During the general strength phase the tempo of exercise performance will generally be slow and controlled. At this stage it is important that the muscles are placed under tension for sufficient time. This principle is known as time under tension (TUT) and is discussed in much greater detail in (chapter 8). Overall the volume of training will be high (lots of sets and reps), and the intensity will be fairly low (heavy loads are not involved). A typical workout may use 2–4 sets of each exercise and 10–15 repetitions.

Specific strength
Having established a baseline of strength qualities and basic control, the priority starts to shift towards directly targeting swimming performance. This is where many programmes come unstuck, often because of a failure to move on to the next stage or doing so inappropriately by trying to recreate swimming with weights.

As already seen, the gym offers the capacity to overload force production in a way that is not possible in the pool. In this phase larger loads can be utilised to develop force production. This will be dominated by pulling movements that reflect the challenge of swimming. The fact that larger loads are being used will naturally mean that the number of repetitions will be fewer than in the previous phase. For example, the athlete who was previously performing 3 sets of 10 chin-ups may now switch to 5 sets of 5 repetitions wearing

a weighted vest to add resistance. Wherever possible the exercise choice should still require body control. This will increase the chances of transfer to pool. As well as having to reduce repetitions, another consequence of introducing more load to the exercise is that the speed of movement will slow down. This is inevitable but the athlete must make every attempt to move the weight with speed. We are developing strength as part of a journey towards power. Performing these exercises with the intent to move quickly will make that journey far easier.

Without delving too deeply into the science of strength training, a significant element of the adaptation to this phase comes from the nervous system. In order to achieve this effectively each set of an exercise should be performed relatively free from fatigue. Therefore, unlike the previous phase, rest intervals will be slightly longer (around 2–3 minutes). The usual feeling of leaving the gym exhausted will also fade somewhat. This often comes very unnaturally to the endurance athlete. The natural positive association with this feeling at the end of every session means that many almost experience a sense of moral guilt if it is not achieved. However this is when we start to learn the difference between exercising and training. If the athlete performs the session in a way that makes them feel good but is not the best way to move forward then they are exercising, not training.

The best recommendation for selecting strength exercises is to make natural progression to the choices used in the general strength phase. These should already have been selected as being suitable in terms of ability to perform them correctly. These can now either have load added to them or a more advanced version used. For example, a triathlete who used partial press-ups in the general phase can now cope with the full version because of strength gains made and the lower number of repetitions required. By following this process there is natural continuity and progression through the programme. This not only helps with progress but is also motivating as advances are made.

There are a great range of set and repetition combinations that can be used during this phase. To some extent these will be determined by the load used. As a rule of thumb, sets of 3–8 repetitions are suitable with a total number not exceeding 25 for each exercise. Popular methods include 3 x 8, 5 x 5 and 6 x 3. In general the stronger the athlete is, the lower the number of repetitions can go. Novice trainers are likely to make the greatest gains towards the higher end of this scale.

Special strength
Finally we come to special strength. Here the gap between swimming and land training is at its smallest. Indeed it may well be that this work is carried out in the pool. We have already seen that resisted swim work can have a positive effect on propulsion power. It is during this final phase that this is most appropriate. For some, land training aimed at swimming propulsion may end at this point to be replaced with the pool equivalent, although land training may still continue to aid reduction of drag and technique.

The qualities to be developed here are those that can directly be used in the swim – namely power and power endurance. Power means that we need speed, and the added weight that was used when developing force previously must be significantly reduced so that explosive actions can be produced. We must also ensure not only that power can be produced but also that it can be produced repeatedly. This requires a delicate balance in the programming of the session.

Explosive exercises performed repeatedly will naturally produce fatigue, and with fatigue comes a loss of speed and power. Therefore the volume and intensity of the session must be carefully managed to ensure that the athlete has to work hard to maintain explosiveness, but that it is still possible. The most effective method is to start with a low number performed very well and gradually increase the repetitions. This will work better than starting high and hoping they will get faster.

One of the most effective tools for this type of work is the medicine ball (as known as a med ball). Unlike traditional weights the ball can be thrown. This is a crucial detail as it means that acceleration can continue through the movement, just as it does through the swimming stroke. Regular gym exercises require deceleration towards the end of the movement and so power cannot be developed optimally. Exercises such as the medicine ball slam are excellent for working on pulling power. Additionally the medicine ball toss will help to develop leg power. Gym exercises may be used during this phase. However the choices must match these movement characteristics: for example, the barbell throw-off represents an explosive variation on the bench press, or a plyometric (clap) press-up may be used. Exercises that utilise jumping such as the jump squat are also ideal for increasing leg power.

4.4 Summary
Enhancing swim performance through strength and conditioning can be achieved through a number of routes that will promote the overall goal of reducing drag and increasing propulsion power. However these gains will not happen by accident or simply doing some general gym work. Rather they must be carefully targeted with an intelligent and considered focus.

005
the bike

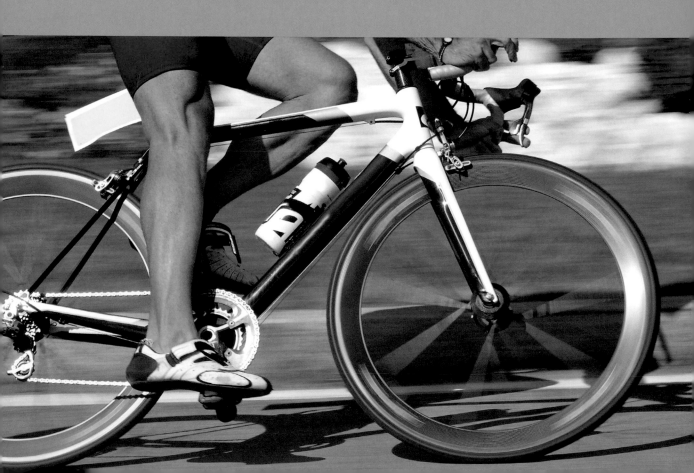

5.1 Introduction

Of the three disciplines that make up triathlon the natural association with S&C is perhaps most obvious in the cycle. Increasing the strength and power of the legs is likely to have a more direct and fruitful transfer to performance in this event than in either the swim or the run. However in the pursuit of excellence there is no room for assumption. We must still be vigilant in ensuring that we are sure of seeing gains by targeting the cycle with strength training. Similarly it is not acceptable to take a lazy approach and simply get a bit stronger and a bit faster. If the aim of triathlon is to be your best then it follows that a rigorous approach to identifying the best strength regime for the best results is essential. In this chapter we look at the evidence supporting S&C for cycling. We also identify the strength qualities required, the adaptations that underpin them and the methods for achieving them.

5.2 The technical basis of S&C for cycling

It may be overly simplistic to look at the swim as a technical event requiring minimal fitness and the bike as the reverse. During flat and downhill cycling the challenge is once again one of drag versus propulsion (obviously the degree of which depends on speed). There are also many modifications in technology and body position which will affect the efficiency of transfer from the body to the bike. That said, powerful legs will produce power on the bike and high speeds. A comprehensive review of the physical qualities that best predict cycling performance in scientific studies revealed the following top three factors:

- Power output at lactate threshold

- Peak power output (ideally a power/weight ratio of at least 5.5 watts/kg)

- The percentage of type I fibres (slow twitch) in the vastus lateralis (quadriceps muscle)

This may surprise many as power is clearly very highly associated with performance in endurance cycling. VO₂ max is notable by its absence. In fact in isolation this is a very poor predictor of performance, and yet it is commonly the primary goal of many triathlete's cycling programmes.

Those involved with sprint cycling on the track need no convincing of the need for strength and power work to be considered a fundamental aspect of training. Those who ply their trade over longer distances on the road sometimes require convincing of the significance to their event. This is surely a changing trend however as a wealth of evidence is now available demonstrating the effects of strength training on endurance cycling. A review of these studies reveals that even in well-trained competitive cyclists gains of 8–10 per cent in time-trial performance are achievable. This is remarkable for a number of reasons. Firstly these gains are typically seen over a period of about 12 weeks and so may represent only the 'tip of the iceberg'. Secondly the training programmes used in the studies are generally very basic and haven't been individualised, because scientific protocol demands they must all perform the same session. Therefore it is reasonable to assume that with more advanced and individualised programming these results could be improved on further. Finally the fact that such large improvements have been achieved in a short period of time in well-trained cyclists is remarkable. In athletes such as these even a 5 per cent improvement over the course of a season would generally be considered very positive progress. When we consider that 10 per cent gains in three months have been repeatedly achieved the value of adding strength to a programme becomes clear.

The case for the importance of strength can also be drawn from the taper. During this period the strength of the quads can be expected to increase in the region of 8 per cent. The same increase is also seen in performance. This is not to claim that gains in performance are entirely the result of strength, but the importance of power is once again evident.

So how do gains in strength affect the way in which an athlete cycles? One of the more interesting changes is a reduction in pedalling cadence during longer rides (while maintaining the same speed). This carries a double benefit: not only does it result in more efficient cycling but also a greater economy during the run. It is this change in efficiency that is the key to enhanced performance. Successful strength-training programmes for cycling always increase maximum power output. Although this absolute maximum is not used during a triathlon the cyclist is now able to work at the same rate, but at a lower percentage of their maximum. As a result the athlete does not feel as if they are working as hard and can either increase the pace or work more efficiently and save energy for the run.

The issue of body weight and cycling also throws up some interesting paradoxes. Any glance through a cycling or triathlon magazine will demonstrate the financial lengths athletes will go to shave a few extra grams from the weight of the bike. All too often the same degree of commitment is not shown when controlling body weight! Of course it is the 'system mass', i.e. the bike plus its rider, that we should be concerned with. This often leads to unfounded fears that resistance training will result in 'bulking up' and the rider losing any gains from strength to added load, which will take its toll during uphill portions of the race. This argument can be countered from two angles. Firstly, and most importantly, the likelihood of

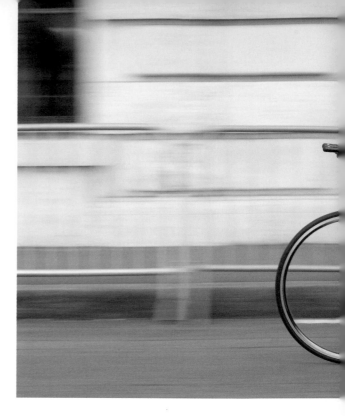

weight gain is incredibly slim. There are a number of reasons behind this:

- Gains in muscle mass require specific protocols, nutritional plans and body type.

- The large volumes of endurance work will block the 'muscle gain pathways' in the body (*see* section 2.2).

- If strength training regimes (rather than bodybuilding) are used then any gains in muscle will come in the form of more densely packed muscles with little weight gain rather than 'pumped up' muscles (*see* figure 1.4).

Much of the gains in strength and power following training are likely to come from changes in the nervous system, particularly following explosive type training. This goes some way to explaining how strength training can enhance performance in the absence of more muscle.

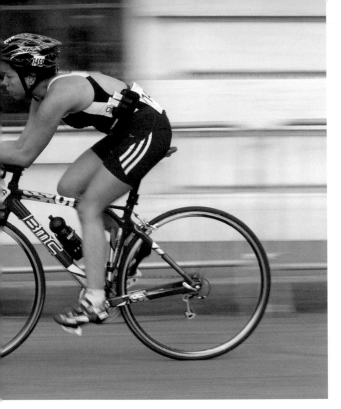

Triathletes will frequently claim that they simply don't have time to add this work. This is generally the result of a fear of letting go of bike work in favour of the gym. To some this suggestion may seem like an S&C coach losing perspective. However the research evidence demonstrates that not only is it possible to drop cycling sessions for weights and still improve performance but that it is also a necessity. Ironically it may even be that part of the value of replacing road work with the gym lies in the strength gains as well as in a reduction of excessive levels of endurance work! In some circles this may sound like the ultimate sacrilege in endurance sport. The evidence however is very strong, and those who break away from old-fashioned training techniques and tradition and allow themselves to be guided by science will gain a crucial edge.

A second element to the debate centres around body composition versus body weight. If despite the factors described above an athlete were to gain a few kilograms of muscle this would add to the system mass and have a negative impact – right? This holds true only if we fail to consider how the body works as a whole. Many triathletes still carry levels of body fat slightly above their optimum. Naturally this also contributes to the system mass. One of the biggest determinants of our basal metabolic rate (the amount of calories our body requires each day before exercise) is the amount of lean body mass. Therefore if we increase lean mass we increase this rate and potentially start to burn off fat at a greater rate. So it is distinctly possible that small gains in muscle may actually change our body composition without affecting body weight.

The scheduling of training sessions is another reason that is often quoted for not including strength work as an integral part of a programme.

So far we have only discussed the role of increased leg strength on performance. This falls into the stereotypical view of a powerful cyclist having an emaciated upper body perched on legs like tree trunks. While the legs are obviously the area we are most concerned with, the trunk and upper body are ignored at our peril. These are crucial to anchor the body so that force can effectively be transferred to the pedals. A very specific type of strength is required in these areas for cycling performance, namely isometric endurance (*see* 'Types of muscle contraction', chapter 1). This essentially means the ability to remain fixed and rigid for long periods of time. Unlike speed or power this is not a quality in which ever-increasing amounts are sought. We simply require an adequate amount to control the force generated by the legs. For some this will come naturally and no additional work is required. However others may find this a limiting factor, and any gains in leg strength are seriously compromised due to 'energy leaks'. These will often be female triathletes and those from a running background who have not historically utilised the upper body to great effect.

5.3 The practical application of S&C to cycling

For a training programme to be successfully transferred to the bike there are several elements that must be considered. Which muscles need to be worked? Which movements should we work them through? What speed of movement works best and how much work should we do?

Figure 5.1 shows the relative contributions of the muscles involved in cycling. The breakdown relates to movements rather than specific muscles and reflects the way in which they should be trained. Of course the figures given are only an approximate guide, as these will vary according to technique, body dimensions, bike set-up and gradient of cycle. That said, it is clear that the most important aspect is knee extension (quads), followed by hip extension (gluteals and hamstrings). Given that these two actions combine to represent around three-quarters of the

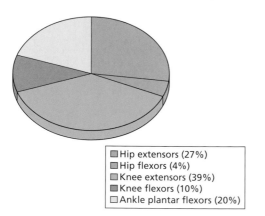

□ Hip extensors (27%)
□ Hip flexors (4%)
□ Knee extensors (39%)
□ Knee flexors (10%)
□ Ankle plantar flexors (20%)

Figure 5.1 Muscle contributions to cycling action.

Ericson (1986), On the biomechanics of cycling. A study of joint and muscle load during exercise on the bicycle ergometer. Scand, J. Rehabil Med Suppl., 16

power production they are clearly a high priority. It is important to recognise that these actions occur together during the pedal action. This means that the greatest transfer will be achieved if we use exercises that also combine simultaneous knee and hip extension. This is also a more efficient way of training, because separate exercises do not need to be used for each action. The calves (ankle plantar flexors) also play an important role, although for practical reasons these are often best trained in isolation. Finally while they do not appear to play a role in power production, the ankle dorsi-flexors are also important. The tibialis anterior (the muscle that runs down the front of the shin) maintains a strong ankle during the back lift of the pedal stroke. Developing strength in this area is also important to maintain a muscle balance with the calf. As with all areas of the body it is important to develop the musculature on both sides of a joint in order to avoid imbalance issues.

Thus the main thrust of a programme for improving leg power for cycling will centre around movements that combine knee and hip extension with supplementary work around the ankle movements. This provides myriad options. The movements can be subdivided into two-legged (bilateral) and one-legged (unilateral). In general bilateral movements tend to be ideal for generating large amounts of force, because there are no issues around balance and so all efforts can be directed towards giving a maximal effort. Unilateral movements on the other hand make up for the lower forces involved by the fact that the movements can be considered more specific to the action of cycling. The most effective approach is generally to utilise bilateral movements early in the season to develop a foundation of strength and progress towards specific unilateral exercises as competition approaches.

High force bilateral exercises

These essentially consist of the dead lift and the squat exercise, and the many variations of both. As we have seen, these exercises allow the athlete to move through the appropriate kinetic chain with potentially high loads. Consequently they are excellent tools for strength development. The skill of the strength and conditioning coach comes in identifying precisely the right movement to suit an athlete's body dimensions and strength requirements.

The dead lift is what is known as a hip dominant exercise. This means that force generation takes place to a greater extent at the hip rather than the knee. Squats on the other hand are known as a knee dominant exercise. The extent to which an exercise is knee or hip dominant is determined by the distance of each joint from the line of the bar (*see* figure 5.2). We have already seen that cycling

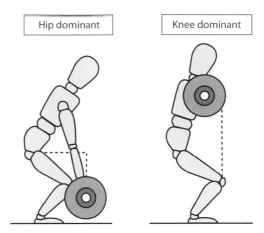

Hip dominant	Knee dominant

Figure 5.2 Knee and hip dominant patterns

is dominated by knee extension over hip extension. As a result squats are generally considered the staple exercise for cycling performance. That is not to say that dead lifts do not have a role to play. Most of us tend to be quite

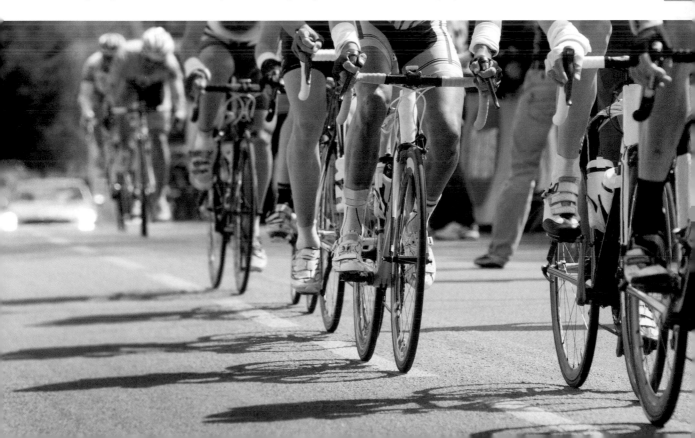

knee dominant in our movement patterns as a result of the adaptations of daily life. This can then be compounded by large volumes of knee dominant cycling. Therefore the dead lift can represent a welcome opportunity to develop strength through the hips and take the load off the knees. The dead lift is also an excellent tool for developing upper body strength and therefore offers additional benefits for athletes who may be lacking in this area.

The squat is a key exercise, which will almost certainly feature in any cycling strength programme, and therefore the variations on the movement warrant some discussion. In general the squat is either performed as a back squat or a front squat (the only major exception is the overhead squat). The terms back and front refer to the position of the bar in relation to the athlete's shoulders. This will have an influence over the

hip–knee balance, but it is often more important to select the lift that suits the athlete best. Many find the front squat somewhat awkward as it requires flexibility of the wrists and lats. Also most people are not able to lift as much in the front squat as the back squat. However those with particularly long thighs may find it hard to perform a back squat correctly (i.e., not leaning forward excessively). It is frequently harder to maintain a healthy back position in the back squat and so those with intervertebral disc problems are advised to use the front squat.

The squat is also a curious enigma in that it is one of the few exercises that is not routinely performed to a full range of motion. Many perform the movement only to a parallel position (thighs parallel to the floor) under the misguided belief that going any deeper is harmful to the knees. This is far from true as in fact the knees become more stable below the parallel position. Through a deeper range of movement the glutes and vatsus medialis also become more involved. These are key muscles in movement control, which many people lack, and so deep squatting is not only safe but also to be encouraged. The absolute depth that one should squat to is hard to define as it depends very much on individual mobility. The short answer is that squats should be developed as deep as good technique allows. There are times when a shorter range is used to allow greater loads to be placed on the bar. However it is strongly suggested that lighter, full range movements are used initially to develop mobility and 'unlock' the athlete's existing strength before adding more to a small range.

The final major option that has not been discussed is the leg press. This is one of the few resistance training machines that is still used regularly by athletes. The leg press uses a similar movement of

Table 5.1	Single-leg exercise categories
Category	**Emphasis**
Single-leg squats (inc. Bulgarian squats and split squats)	Greatest potential for strength development Several variations that allow for development of range of movement and control
Lunges	Balance of strength and control development A large number of variations that can be used to target different aspects of the hip and leg musculature
Step-ups	Most specific movement pattern to cycling, which mimics the downward thrust on the crank Excellent choice for challenging control of the trunk, hips, knees and ankles Ability to load heavily may be restricted

the hips and knees to squatting patterns but can generally be loaded to a greater extent as the need for control is removed. From this perspective it is an excellent choice as the athlete's strength levels can be challenged to maximal levels without the need to develop technique and control. It could certainly be argued that this is a good fit for cycling strength training as the pedals and crank also control the gross movement pattern. Others would argue that developing athleticism is also important. This will include control of the hips, knees and ankles and strengthening the back and trunk. In the case of the triathlete, rather than the pure cyclist, these are certainly important qualities. For the triathlete who is a novice strength trainer it may be best to use lighter squats and dead lifts to develop athleticism and build a platform of technique for future training while using the leg press to build strength in the meantime. More advanced trainers who are able to perform heavy squats with good technique are lucky enough to be able to develop strength and athleticism simultaneously.

Unilateral leg exercises

There are three main categories of single-leg exercise that are likely to be used to develop cycling strength, each of which brings its own particular emphasis (*see* table 5.1). The single-leg squat is possibly the best choice for developing single-leg strength. Exercises such as the Bulgarian squat and the split squat fall into this category and allow high levels of load and strength development. The single-leg squat off a box and pistols are also excellent movements that use body weight as the main form of resistance. The lunge is a very versatile exercise, although it is generally not loaded particularly heavily. Of the many variations the reverse lunge is a much ignored but very effective tool. Finally step-ups provide an obvious choice owing to the similarity of the movement to the pedalling action. Once again though the demand for control is high if these are to be performed correctly. Therefore relying on them too heavily is likely to mean major compromises in strength development.

Explosive leg exercises

It must always be remembered that the ultimate aim of work directed towards increased cycling power is power itself. This means that force is produced rapidly. As a result it is important to include some explosive work in the strength programme. Most traditional gym exercises do not lend themselves to explosive work as the weight needs to be decelerated towards the end of the movement. The natural answer to this issue is jumping-based exercises, which are inherently explosive. These can be manipulated to be either high or low load biased: for example, bodyweight jumps will maximise explosiveness with a light load; moderate loadings can be achieved with medicine ball throwing exercises, whereas the whole spectrum of loads can be worked with jump squats.

As well as jumping exercises, the Olympic lifts (i.e., cleans and snatches) are very popular power-development tools that feature in virtually every text on strength and conditioning. These are certainly very effective for developing power when used correctly. The power outputs achieved in these lifts generally exceed all other options including jump squats. However the task of performing them correctly is not a simple one. Developing the technique to a level that is both safe and effective requires a great deal of practice and expert tuition. As a result it is suggested that the vast majority of triathletes are likely to be able to use their training time more effectively by using more simplistic techniques. For those who are keen to utilise the Olympic lifts the most effective approach may be to use teaching drills to develop the skills and mobility as part of a warm-up. This can be done in tandem with other power-development methods until the athlete has developed sufficient technical ability to perform loaded Olympic lifts for power development.

The selection of loading for explosive exercises is an important element that must be considered. By their nature these exercises must be performed with speed. Therefore the weight that is used must be somewhere comfortably below the maximum that can be lifted. The ideal load is a matter of some debate. Many coaches seek to use the load that produces the maximal mechanical power output. This typically occurs at loads of 40–50 per cent of the one-repetition maximum for a given exercise (with the exception of Olympic lifts where it is closer to 85–90 per cent). Alternatively a load can be used to target high-load power or low-load power depending on the needs of the athlete. For example, a small quick athlete who lacks strength is likely to be better suited to high-load power work that will target the force element of force x velocity, which makes up power. On the other hand an athlete who is very strong but not particularly explosive may benefit most from working on low-load power, which will emphasise the speed component of power. The most important factor to remember is that a maximal effort to move the weight as fast as possible must be made. This intent to move the weight quickly is actually more important than the result itself. Indeed, as has been shown, attempting to move very heavy loads quickly improves power even if the weight ends up moving only very slowly.

Exercises for the calf and ankle

Most of the strength exercises described so far include movements of the hips and knees, which as we have seen are the main driving forces in cycling power. However it would be foolish to ignore the 20 per cent contribution made by the calves to pedal power. A brief glance at the lower leg of most top cyclists also tells us that this is a pretty important area.

When it comes to explosive work the ankle is pretty well catered for by the jumping movements already discussed. Therefore we are primarily concerned with developing strength in the muscle. This is a relatively straightforward process as the movement of plantar flexion (pointing the toes) is a fairly simple one. Therefore all of the exercises for this movement will be variations on the calf raise exercise. The movement is produced by the two calf muscles – gastrocnemius and soleus. In order to target both effectively it is important to perform some movements with a straight leg (for gastrocnemius) and some with a bend in the knee (for soleus). On this occasion machines such as the leg press (with straight legs) or the calf raise are just as beneficial as bodyweight or free-weight exercises. These are actually useful tools as the mechanics of the calf allow large loads to be lifted, and machines may remove the danger of difficult balancing acts.

Finally as already discussed, we must also develop the tibialis anterior (which runs along the outside of the shin) in order to balance the development of the calf and allow for a strong ankle during the backstroke. Once again training the action of dorsi-flexion (lifting toes towards the shin) is a relatively straightforward one. This can be achieved though tib ant raises (see chapter 9) or through the use of resistance bands (see chapter 8). These are ideal for general development of the muscle and for retaining balance in the lower leg.

Exercises for the upper body and trunk

In general those who lack sufficient upper body strength for optimal cycling performance will also lack general upper body strength. An athlete with good general strength and sufficient size in their upper body simply needs to practise cycling techniques and riding different gradients in order to start to use this more effectively. That is not to say that we cannot try to fill our gym work with exercises that will potentially have a greater carry

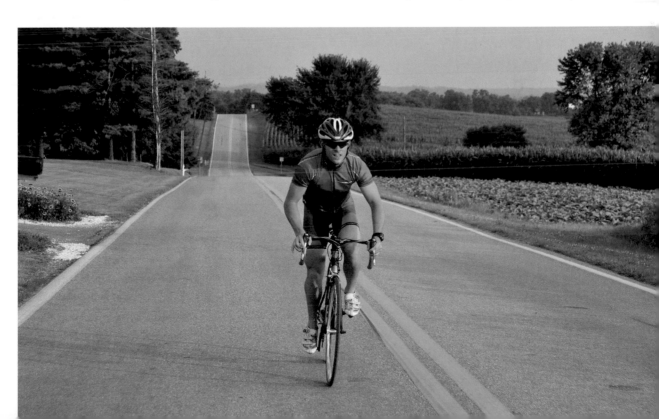

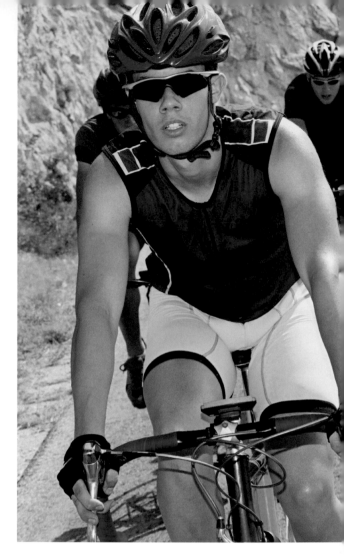

over to cycling. The key thing to remember is that the strength of the upper body must be matched by the trunk. Exercises that support the trunk such as the bench press allow an imbalance to develop and the trunk starts to become a weak link.

We must also keep sight of the fact that the way in which we train for one discipline will also impact on the other two. The choices we have presented for developing strength in the swim are also good options for the challenge of the bike (*see* table 4.2). This is certainly true during general winter training. For those with greater levels of S&C experience and as the competitive season approaches it is possible to adapt these generic exercises to make them somewhat more specific to cycling power (*see* table 5.2). This also adds some variety to maintain interest and avoid plateaux. As ever though, the athlete should only progress to these once competency has been achieved in the simplest form of the exercise.

The trunk can be trained effectively by using these types of exercises, but there is also value in adding additional trunk-specific work where time allows. Once again this should be focused on preventing movement around the trunk rather than generating it. The plank is a mainstay of many triathletes' training programmes and its position there is well justified. However a few notes of caution should be exercised. If we are aiming to target the trunk/ abdomen then it is vital that the arms, chest and

shoulders are kept relaxed. It is a common sight to see a hunched upper back and hands gripped with tension as an athlete seeks to last a little longer by taking the strain through the wrong areas. If this cannot be prevented then an easier version of the

Table 5.2	Some cycling upper body options		
Category	Basic option	Variation 1	Variation 2
Presses	Press-up	Deep weighted press-ups	Single-arm press-ups
Pulls	Inverse pulls	Single-arm bent-over row	Pull-ups

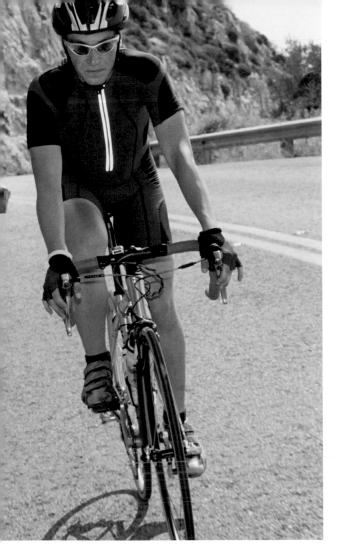

example, a three-point plank (two legs and one arm, or vice versa) will achieve this perfectly. Other choices such as aleknas, dead bugs and leg raises are also ideal.

5.4 Periodisation and progression of cycle strength

Some riders feel that the gym is not needed for them to put strength in their legs. Instead they believe that they can make excellent gains in a more specific manner through working tough hills or going through a hard session on a big chain ring. These are indeed excellent methods of developing specific strength for cycling. The ability to change the forces applied for a given speed through the use of the gears is one of the unique features of the bike and makes it a much more adaptable tool. So does that mean the gym is redundant? Not at all. The gym still has an even greater capacity to overload force, which means that if we want to improve maximum strength then this is still the best option. The gym also offers the ability to work in different ways. As we have seen, most cyclists already do enough cycling so the opportunity to develop with different tools is often more powerful. Finally the gym provides a chance to redress any muscular imbalances or areas of weakness that are exacerbated by further cycling.

So which option should we go for? The answer is both, with a shift through the year from general to specific. By using the winter to get the body in balance, target weak areas and develop basic physical qualities such as maximum strength the triathlete is then in a great position to start to transfer these gains through the spring. This will see a general shift towards more explosive work followed by a much greater reliance on bike strength sessions as the competitive season approaches (*see* chapter 7 for more on periodisation).

exercise needs to be used. The next point regards how long to go for. It should not be the aim to perform an everlasting plank! The endurance element comes from the bike, the strength element comes from the gym. Therefore once a plank of 60+ seconds can be performed comfortably with good technique it is time to introduce more advanced variations. One way of achieving this is to add a small weight across the hips. Another is to reduce the number of points-of-contact with the floor. The latter of these may be the preferred choice as it replicates the diagonal forces that are transferred across the body during cycling (as well as swimming and running for that matter). For

65

006
the run

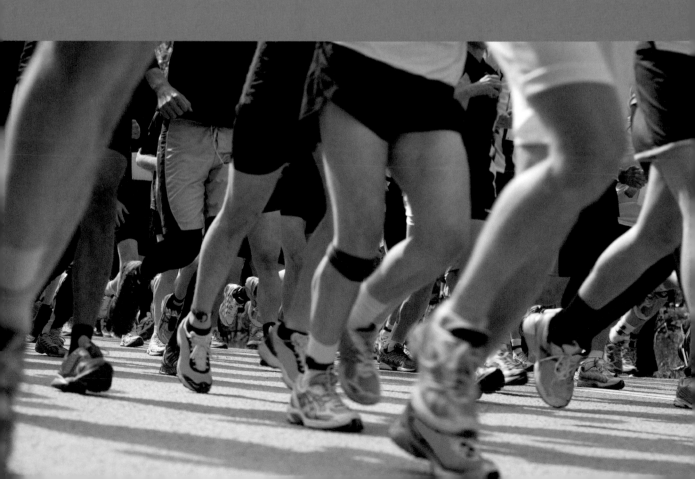

6.1 Introduction

Running is a curious term as it describes many forms of movement that often have little in common! The complex interplay between limbs, torso and the ground is a highly sophisticated mechanical operation, which doesn't happen by chance. Therefore it is fair to say that, while almost everyone can run, very few of us can really run. Improving our technical ability in the run is one of the most potent, yet neglected, ways of increasing speed and efficiency and bringing down times. Therefore it should come as no surprise that S&C for endurance running is concerned firstly with improving the quality of our movement and secondly with the quantity.

Many triathlon books and magazines acknowledge the fact that running technique is important and try to help athletes by giving general advice on its technique. In the main though this is entirely useless, because the movements and postures displayed when we run are a result of our physical structures, strengths and weaknesses. An athlete could study the technique of a top runner for years, but without the requisite conditioning would still not be able to run to the same excellent standard. It is a common sight to see joggers in the street slumped forwards, arms flailing and knees collapsing. These people do not run that way because they have misunderstood the technical model. They run that way because these are the positions their bodies naturally select.

The antithesis of the plodding, labouring jogger in the street is the majestic Kenyan. It is often remarked that these runners look effortless – this is not an illusion. By holding correct form the efficient runner can reuse elastic energy so they literally bounce along the ground. So how does the plodding jogger start to become more like the majestic Kenyan? Certainly not by practising more plodding! The answer lies in S&C, yet requires an innate understanding of both running mechanics and the S&C tools that are used. To improve technique and efficiency it is generally necessary to get stronger. Here though we are talking very much of postural strength, which is a product of both the strength of the muscles involved and the coordination and skill to use this strength in the correct sequences. With well-directed training everyone can achieve this, but it will not happen by chance or through thrown-together training programmes.

6.2 The technical basis of S&C for running

It has been stated throughout this book that in order to justify its place in a busy training schedule all S&C interventions should be backed up by evidence rather than built on assumption. Therefore we should begin by examining the scientific evidence and the reasons behind it.

Most of the studies into the effects of S&C on endurance running have been based around explosive-strength training. This itself is rather surprising as this probably represents the 'icing on the cake' rather than the first area to focus on. Nonetheless these studies have consistently demonstrated that this type of training improves running economy. This may surprise many as some would assume that this type of work would aid sprinting but have little effect on distance economy. The mechanisms behind these improvements come from several potential sources, the significance of which will depend somewhat on the make-up of the individual. These include increased muscular power, neuromuscular control and improved reactive strength. Most notably they do not include aerobic factors such as VO_2 max. Therefore this represents an area of potential improvement which is 'untapped' by conventional endurance training, the benefits of which will inevitably reduce as the rule of diminishing returns kicks in (*see* section 2.2).

This improvement in running economy translates to improved times as runners are able to produce more speed without increasing the relative intensity. For example, a 5 per cent reduction in 5km race performance has been achieved with just eight weeks of weight training, even in highly trained runners who have less room for improvement. The results of many of the recent scientific studies are summarised in table 6.1.

These benefits alone are good justification for using S&C to improve running performance. However this use of explosive lifting may be only the tip of the iceberg. Increasing the power that the legs can produce is obviously going to help improve running power. However efficient running involves highly technical biomechanics. If an S&C programme does not address these first then unless the athlete is already very technically proficient only a small percentage of the power gained will be transferred into running power.

The stretch shortening cycle and elastic running efficiency

Perfect technical running is not an achievable goal for the vast majority of triathletes. In fact most elite triathletes and even endurance track athletes have technical deficiencies, which take them away from the perfect technical model, and yet still produce superb performances. The key is not to achieve perfection but to hit certain key 'shapes' that allow the body to move efficiently.

We will look at these key positions shortly, but first it is necessary to understand why these shapes are important. The answer lies in a phenomenon known as the stretch shortening cycle. This is the key to elastic energy and efficient running. Our tendons (tissue that joins muscle to bones) have good elastic properties. This means that they have the potential to stretch and then rapidly recoil to return energy. The most important of these tendons with respect to running are the Achilles tendon, which connects the calf to the heel, and the patella tendon, which attaches the quadriceps muscles to the front of the shin. When the foot strikes the floor the runner has the potential to use this elastic recoil to spring back off the ground with relative ease, thus making for efficient movement. Indeed it has been estimated that up to 60 per cent energy is provided by elastic recoil in the best runners. This seemingly 'free energy' comes with a conditional clause.

The 'reusable energy' provided by the stretch shortening cycle is only available for a limited, brief period of time – just a few hundred milliseconds – and the energy potential is reduced the longer the foot is in contact with the ground. Furthermore the elastic potential can be realised only if there is 'active tension' in the muscle. For example, if the muscles around the ankle are relaxed on foot strike then the ankle will simply bend as the weight of the body forces it toward the shin. Similarly if the quads and hamstrings are relaxed then the knee will simply give way and any potential for recoil is lost. Avoiding movement in these key joints during foot strike is known as mechanical stiffness and is one of the key goals of plyometric training (*see* practical application below). This means that the muscles of both sides of the joint co-contract and prevent movement at the joint. The forces are then transferred to the tendons and their elastic properties can be unlocked.

Does this mean that runners should aim to run with these muscles tensed at all times then? Of

Table 6.1	Summary of strength training and running economy research						
Authors	Subject description	Age (Y)	Resistance training, type and duration	Description of treatment and control groups	Results	Improvement (%)	PEDro Scale (32) score (max = 10)
Paavolainen et al.	18 elite male distance runners; Vo_2max = 68 ml kg⁻¹·min⁻¹	20–30	Plyometric training 9 wk	CT = 68% ET, 32% sport-specific plyometric training; ET = 97% ET, 3% sport-specific plyometric training	Decreased 5k run time in CT; improved RE in CT	3.1 (5K); 8.1 (RE)	5
Spurrs et al.	17 male distance runners; Vo_2max = 57 ml kg⁻¹·min⁻¹	n/a	Plyometric training 6 wk	CT = concurrent plyometric training (two sessions per week for 3 weeks then three sessions per week for 3 weeks) and normal ET; ET = continued normal training	Decreased 3K run time in CT improved RE in CT	2.7 (3K) 4–7 (RE)	6
Mikkola et al.	18 male, 7 female distance runners; Vo_2max = 62 ml kg⁻¹·min⁻¹	16–18	Plyometric training 8 wk	CT = 81% endurance and supplemental training, 19% sport-specific explosive strength training; ET = 96% endurance and supplemental training, 4% sport-specific explosive strength training	No Δ RE or Vo_2max increased anaerobic and selective neuromuscular performance in CT	3	5
Saunders et al.	15 elite male distance runners; Vo_2max = 68–70 ml kg⁻¹·min⁻¹	20–30	Plyometric training 9 wk	CT = concurrent plyometric training (3 sessions per week) and normal ET	Improved RE in CT	4.1	6
Millet et al.	15 elite male triathletes; Vo_2max = 67–69 ml kg⁻¹·min⁻¹	18–30	Heavy weight training 1.4 wk	CT = concurrent HWT (lower limb, two sessions per week) and consistent, supervised aerobic training; ET = consistent, supervised aerobic training	Improved RE in CT	5.3	6
Average			9.2 wk			4.5	5.6

CT= concurrent resistance and endurance training; ET= endurance training; HWT= heavy weight training; RE= running economy

Source: Yamamoto 2008

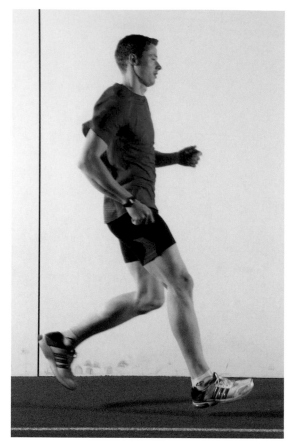

Figure 6.1a Tony Hip (toe–knee–hip) running style

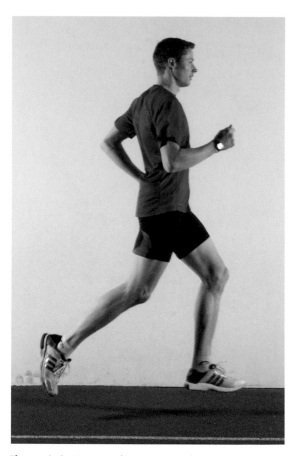

Figure 6.1b Hipneeto (hip–knee–toe) running style

course not. Relaxation is also critical for fluid and smooth movement. The key is to develop the complex, automatic coordination required to run with great relaxation yet be able to instantaneously produce great tension in the correct areas with precision timing. In running this is known as an active foot strike. This may sound intimidatingly complex but can be developed with relatively simple methods (*see* section 6.3).

Key positions for efficient running

So what are the key positions and how do they help promote efficiency? The best way I have heard

this explained was by a colleague and friend who is also a top athletics coach with an excellent understanding of human movement. When analysing my running style he told me he thought I ran like a make-believe English runner who he called Tony Hip (toe–knee–hip). This referred to the order in which I moved the body parts when running (*see* figure 6.1a). Instead he told me he wanted me to run like a Kenyan runner who he called Hipneeto (hip–knee–toe) (*see* figure 6.1b).

The vast majority of us run in the toe–knee–hip style, particularly during longer, slower runs.

This promotes what is known as rear side mechanics as opposed to front side mechanics, which is achieved through the hip–knee–toe running. These terms refer to where the running cycle occurs in relation to the mid-line of the body.

The most crucial point during hip–knee–toe running, or front side mechanics, is immediately after toe-off (the moment the foot leaves the ground). This point represents a crossroads for the rest of the running cycle. During front side running the hip is immediately flexed at the same time as the knee. This brings the free leg (swing leg) through rapidly. On the other hand, rear side running generally sees the foot leave the floor without the hip flexing. The foot then 'floats' out behind the runner, slowly drifting up towards the backside. All the while this is happening the opposite foot is on the ground and is itself approaching the time of toe-off. The front side runner is in a good position as the legs have crossed early and the thigh has been lifted. This puts the runner in a great position to place the foot deliberately on the ground for an active foot strike, which can take advantage of the stretch shortening cycle. He can also place his foot downwards and underneath his hips to minimise the braking forces. Sadly though our rear side runner, Tony Hip, has only just brought his leg through. Rather than actively placing the foot the need for balance means that the foot simply 'splats' on to the ground with little or no active tension. This means there is little potential for elastic energy and the ground contact will be long. The foot will often land significantly in front of the body as well and will thus brake the runner and kill their existing speed! The degree to which front side running is expressed will depend on the speed of the runner. During sprinting the thigh will come close to parallel to the ground. Clearly this is not sustainable during the final leg of an Ironman race. However the same patterns are used, just to a lesser degree.

Another area of some significant debate is that of the foot strike (the position of the foot when it contacts the ground). Many modern coaches believe that a mid-foot strike is optimal as, theoretically at least, this should allow the runner to benefit from the natural mechanics of the foot. The foot is actually a surprisingly complex mechanical design, which is able to control and return force for increased efficiency. By initially landing on the heel it is believed that the runner may not be able to take advantage of this, and such an action also significantly reduces the stretch potential of the Achilles tendon. On the other hand, coaches of the opposite view cite the fact that there is still little direct evidence of a performance-enhancement effect when switching to a mid-foot strike. Furthermore it is claimed that making this move can lead to increased stress around the foot and ankle and increased risk of injury. So who is right? The answer is resoundingly unclear. While the theory regarding greater performance with a mid-foot strike is sound there is no evidence to show that this actually works. Studies have shown that top runners are split between the heel and mid-foot strike, and this does not appear to differentiate between performance. We would suggest that deliberately focusing on the foot position and consciously trying to land on the mid-foot is a bad idea. Instead if you focus on the mechanics of the hip the foot will naturally alter its position in a way that is much more likely to be technically correct. What's more is that these changes will happen gradually as technique slowly moves towards a more front side bias. This gradual change will allow the elastic structures of the foot such as the plantar fascia and Achilles tendon time to adjust to the new demands being placed on them. If the change is made too rapidly the chance of injury is very high and any potential advantage is lost to time on the physio bed. If the foot is placed in the right position (i.e., under the hip rather than in front) then the optimal foot strike should look after itself. Therefore once again hip–knee–toe beats toe–knee–hip.

Regardless of your foot strike one area that cannot be disputed is the importance of good feet. As already learned, the foot is a well-designed mechanical structure. However for many of us they are more like dead slabs of flesh hanging from the end of our shins! This is due to years of neglect and poor footwear. When we consider that our only opportunity to produce speed is via the feet and their contact with the ground this becomes a concern. The other advantage to good foot mechanics is the potential to dissipate and control forces. When this is not done effectively excessive force must be tolerated by other joints and structures that are less suitable for taking them. Given that forces several times our body weight must be absorbed each step we take it is crucial that this is avoided. Therefore a good foot conditioning routine is a must for the running component of a triathlete's training regime.

The potential to discuss the minutiae of every aspect of running technique is almost limitless. However there is neither the capacity nor need to discuss this level of detail in this book. By gaining an understanding of the critical shapes outlined above, combined with the drilling and training techniques below, triathletes of all levels will be able to maximise their potential. In general I have found that giving the body the capacity to achieve the correct positions is more effective than teaching the brain. However in order that athletes may feel they know what they are aiming for, a summary of the tenets of good technique are described in table 6.2.

In summary it is important that an S&C programme first addresses a runner's mechanics in order to make efficient use of their existing strength and power and to take advantage of the potential for elastic energy. Once this has been achieved then the focus can turn towards developing reactive strength and further gains in strength and power to enhance performance.

Table 6.2	The basics of running technique
Area	**Technical goals**
General	Tall relaxed posture with hips held high
Upper body	Shoulders loose with a small amount of rotation
	Elbow angle not critical but should have minimal forward travel in front of body with some movement behind torso
	Avoid elbows flaring or excessive rotation
Hips and lower body	Pelvis in athlete's own neutral (i.e., same as in standing)
	Hip–knee–toe running action
	Neutral/dorsi flexed ankle at foot strike and through swing phase

6.3 The practical application of S&C to running

As we have seen, the focus of S&C for enhancing running performance can be divided into three main areas: muscle conditioning to improve technique; muscle coordination to improve technique and efficiency; and strength qualities such as force, power and reactive strength. We will now further examine the first two of these, which are directed toward the same goal.

Muscular conditioning and coordination

We should be very clear right from the outset that strengthening a muscle in isolation will not miraculously result in changes in running technique. This is a common mistake that many less well-informed physiotherapists and trainers make. The classic example of this comes from the glutes. Because of common movement dysfunctions such as lower crossed syndrome (*see* figure 3.2) underactive glutes are a commonly diagnosed problem. This can lead to all sorts of problems with running technique. However simple glute exercises on a mat alone will not help, even though strengthening the glutes is an important part of the process towards ultimately solving the problem if the muscle is fundamentally weak.

The exercises that we can potentially use to improve technique, range from very simple ones that isolate small movements to whole body exercises that target gross postures. In general the latter is more effective as multiple areas can be targeted and the potential for transfer is greater due to the coordinated nature of the movement. However if there is a particular area of weakness good technique may not be achievable, and so these weak areas must be worked in isolation before being incorporated into larger movements.

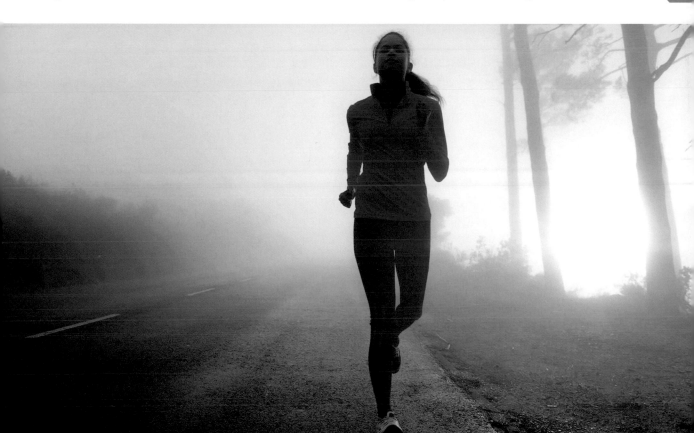

The trunk

The muscles and movements that are most important for improving running technique generally focus around the pelvis and the trunk. If these are controlled optimally then much of the technique in the legs will often take care of itself. Therefore our discussion should start at the centre of the body and move out.

On the most simplistic level the conditioning programme will begin with strengthening the muscles of the trunk in floor-based exercises. These same movements may also have a place in an athlete's programme as part of a prehab routine (see chapter 3). The abdominal exercises should generally be focused on exercises that work to prevent movement (such as the plank and aleknas) rather than more old-fashioned exercises such as sit-ups. The reason these exercises are important is that they aid our ability to control the position of the pelvis and trunk during running. This must be remembered at all times, as good technique is paramount. If technique is sloppy or the exercise level is too advanced the athlete may still work the muscles but will not be practising the control required during running. Often it is control rather than strength that is the limiting factor. A good test for this is the Superman exercise. Performing this movement slowly and quadruped (on all fours) helps to develop a sense of awareness and control around the trunk. These qualities of strength and control must always be developed in tandem as one without the other is useless.

While these exercises form the main component of the trunk conditioning programme the principles of trunk control carry over into the larger movements such as squat and lunge patterns. Once again performing these movements with the view that they are simply 'leg exercises' grossly misses the point and removes much of the potential benefit. In these exercises athletes often arch their backs in order to stabilise the spine. This strategy is no good for the triathlete as it puts the pelvis in a poor position. Ideally the muscles of the abdomen and lower back work together in a co-contraction. This keeps the pelvis in its natural position and optimises the stability of the spine. It is for these reasons that good technique with a light weight (or no weight at all) always beats a heavy bar with suboptimal technique. Once an adequate level of strength has been achieved along with basic control in mat exercise, whole body movements such as these are critical for transfer to the demands of running. It is this vital integration stage that is often missing from programmes and the reason for their subsequent failure to affect technique. The third stage comes from running drills (see below).

The hips

The muscles of the hips (the glutes) play a key role in holding good form and technique during running. Once again training this area can include basic exercises to make the muscles stronger right through to large whole body exercises that incorporate this strength into a gross movement pattern.

The glutes are primarily responsible for hip extension (pulling the thigh backwards). During running this also helps to keep the hips in a 'high position'. Most recreational runners tend to run in a position that athletics coaches call 'sitting down'. This puts the athlete in a poor position to take advantage of the elastic qualities of the hamstrings and can shorten the stride. However holding the high position requires a good level of conditioning and technique.

The glutes are also responsible for hip abduction (lifting the leg outwards). During the running action the muscle uses its hip abduction component to keep the hips level and avoid 'kicking out' to the side. During the most basic isolation exercises though we simply need to make sure that the muscles are challenged in both these tasks. It is also important the glutes are actually worked. Many individuals find it hard to fire their glutes effectively. If this is the case it is vital that the correct level of exercise is selected. It should be possible to feel the muscle working, either by the athlete feeling the effort or a coach feeling tension in the muscle. Quite often an exercise of too hard a level is chosen and the underactive glutes must be helped out by the hamstrings. If this is the case then the dysfunctional pattern of dominant hamstrings and underactive glutes will simply be exacerbated. Table 6.3 gives examples of glute exercises and levels of progression.

Hip dominant squatting patterns and dead lifts are an excellent method of improving the hip extension strength of the glutes during a whole body movement. It is important to realise that the amount of glute activity also increases as the squat becomes deeper. This is a point often missed by novice trainers who restrict themselves to shallow squats in the mistaken belief that this mirrors the small range of movement seen during running. However by utilising the fullest range of movement that can be performed with good technique it is possible to hit the glutes to the fullest extent.

The Neutral Pelvis and Pelvic Control

Many physiotherapists and trainers often talk of a 'neutral pelvis'. This refers to the amount of forward rotation and essentially means the mid-position. This can be difficult to judge during running as different athletes have different natural alignments. Perhaps it is more important not which position the pelvis is in, but that the athlete has control. Many sprinters naturally have a lordotic posture (pelvis tilted forwards), but providing the athlete is not collapsing into this position good technique can still be maintained.

The most effective method of challenging the ability of the glutes to keep the hips stable laterally and not kick out is through single-leg patterns. For example, single-leg squats, lunges and step-ups all provide a challenge. All of these are relatively slow and controlled movements. This is desirable for allowing the athlete time to control the movement and also places the muscle under tension for long durations that will aid strength development. This does not reflect what happens during running though, as the body only has a few hundred milliseconds on each foot strike to stabilise the hips. Once again this is why the third level of conditioning is required in the form of drills and low-level plyometrics.

Table 6.3	Glute exercise options		
	Basic	Intermediate	Advanced
Hip extension	Fire hydrants	Glute bridge	Single-leg glute bridge
Hip abduction	Clam shells	Side lying leg raise	Band walks

The feet

We have already seen that the foot has a complex mechanical structure that can aid the efficiency of running and help to dissipate forces to reduce the strain on the rest of the body. Much has been made of the concept of barefoot running in the popular press in recent years. This is intended to help utilise the foot to its natural design. Ironically this has resulted in a generation of 'barefoot running shoes'. While this may be the ultimate example of every problem looking like a nail if the only tool you have is a hammer it demonstrates the importance of feet. While it is a matter of personal opinion we would suggest the best solution is to perform dedicated foot conditioning sessions and run in regular trainers. This offers the best of both worlds as it allows the athlete to use the support of the trainer with well-conditioned feet.

There is no difference between injury prevention and performance-enhancing work for the feet. Therefore the foot conditioning routine outlined in chapter 3 provides a good routine for maintaining foot and ankle health.

Global posture

Having good global posture, i.e., good balance and alignment across the major joints, is important to provide a foundation for good technique. If the athlete does not have good posture to begin with there will always be limitations to running technique. This then needs to be extended to dynamic posture. This means having the strength and balance to maintain a balanced posture during movement. The potential for improvements in global posture through weight training is frequently overlooked by novice coaches and athletes. Far too often weight training is viewed simply as a method of getting stronger or bigger. However whole body barbell exercises are extremely powerful tools for making positive changes to the quality of an athlete's movement. By focusing on good technique and range of movement rather than simply the weight on the bar great gains can be made. Therefore squatting and lunge patterns once again represent an ideal tool for improving running mechanics, or at least the capacity to support good mechanics. The alternative of course is to try to address each aspect of posture individually. While this may occasionally be necessary if there is a significant problem it is generally a very time-consuming approach. What's more it is generally less effective at improving global posture, because unlike whole body methods the muscles and joints are not required to correct themselves in a coordinated pattern.

As you can see, the best practice approach to developing the raw material to underpin good running technique is through the use of whole body squat and lunge patterns, supplemented with well-selected isolated conditioning exercises to develop targeted areas of weakness. However in order to start to have a positive impact on technique, and ultimately performance, we must start to turn this raw material into specific conditioning.

Drills and running exercises

If general training helps to build the raw material for good running technique then the running drills provide the craft to turn them into the finished article. These exercises are a broad category that can include traditional running drills, hurdle drills and high-speed running. These forms of training work through two mechanisms. Firstly they allow us to work through the movement patterns, or elements of the pattern, which relate to good running technique. This is a form of skill training and also helps to teach the body to incorporate new-found strength into the complex whole body movements of running. Secondly the training also provides another means to strengthen the relevant muscles. The intensity of work on a given muscle group is generally far less than one may feel when working in an isolation exercise. However what is lost in intensity is more than made up for in specificity. Because the value in these exercises lies in the movement patterns they are performed in it is first important to learn to perform them with excellent technique. Once this is possible then we can focus on performing them with excellent technique for longer.

Running drills

There are an almost unlimited number of running drills that athletics coaches can use, although these can be broken down into broad themes. The key to running drills is to understand that they are primarily training the nervous system. As a result they must be handled with great care, as poor technique will result in teaching the body poor patterns, not to mention wasting time. If you do not have access to an experienced and competent athletics or S&C coach it may be most sensible to focus on becoming really good at a handful of simple drills rather than lots of drills that are performed with several flaws. While each running drill is designed to target specific technical aspects of running technique there are a number of core principles that should apply to all drills:

- **Engage in 'deliberate practice':** If we are to make real gains in developing skill it is critical to be fully engaged and focused on the task in hand. When we are in this optimal zone the body starts to increase the amount of myelin produced. This is a substance that 'hardwires' the coordination patterns from the nervous system to develop complex and refined skills (for more on this fascinating subject see *Talent Code* by Daniel Coyle). The positions two athletes produce may look very similar, but if one is truly focused on gaining greater control

of their body and the other is not then their rate of progression will be very different. Even if perfection has been achieved the athlete should still strive further to improve.

- **Move with the 'flow' at all times:** This is an absolutely critical concept which if not understood will mean that, no matter how perfect the shapes an athlete makes, they will never truly teach the muscles to work in the complex symphony required for efficient running. Flow means that the athlete is at once tall, strong and stable yet at the same time utterly relaxed and effortless. The best examples of this can often be seen in top sprinters who are clear of the field and moving seemingly effortlessly. These runners are still having to produce huge forces to achieve and maintain these speeds, but at the same time remain free from tension. In contrast the athletes trailing them are often tight and rigid with tension in their desperation to catch them, and as a result the gap between them can only widen. When being coached in drills the simple cue of 'flow' can often be highly effective in reminding the athlete to relax. If we are engaging in deliberate practice it is often human nature to start to tense up as we concentrate so hard on achieving perfect technique.

- **Posture:** Although each running drill has its own specific technical focus, the one constant throughout all drills and exercises should be posture. This can often be forgotten when the focus is placed too closely on one area of technique. It is important to remember that in order to claim to have good technique the whole body must be doing the right thing, not just the legs! Posture gives us the foundation for this technique. Therefore if you are watching your own or another triathlete's technique, always start with posture.

- **Start with low volumes and build:** When developing technique it is important that we do not increase the volume until we have nailed the technique over a short distance. Ignoring this principle will simply develop the ability to maintain poor technique! All drills should start very simply over a short distance and gradually expand. Do not worry about the speed along the ground either. Remember, this is not running, it is technique work and a desire to move quickly from A to B is an easy way to destroy technique.

Running drills vary in their difficulty, which is mainly determined by the speed at which they are performed. Most drills start with a walking or marching variation. This allows the body plenty of time to find, adjust and correct its positions and learn how it 'feels' to make the correct shapes. These are often expanded into skips. They are performed more quickly and start to develop the rhythm and timings required during running. Finally the drills are expanded into runs (although a long way off top speed). Even at submaximal paces, there is no time to make adjustments if the correct positions are not achieved immediately. Therefore it is unwise to progress before excellent technique has been achieved in walking and skipping drills. Remember, it is far better to perform a walk with good technique than a march with bad. Chapter 11 describes a number of drills that can be used to this end.

Hurdle drills
Visit any athletics track and you are almost guaranteed to see someone trackside walking over hurdles or skipping through them with the rhythm of a dancer. To the uninitiated these may seem

exclusive property of the hurdlers, yet this couldn't be further from the truth. If running drills are mainly aimed at developing specific technique, hurdle drills are fantastic for improving posture and control. By stepping over the high hurdles and pushing our bodies through ranges of movement unfamiliar in daily life, huge gains can be made in mobility and control.

There is one small problem. For many, the high hurdles of the track are far too big, even on the lowest setting. Athletes often ignore this and attempt to perform the drills regardless. Naturally this results is some horrible-looking postures and techniques. The body is forced to find 'other ways' of getting over the hurdle and so when there is no more room for the hips to move the lower back flexes, the shoulders round and the head pokes forwards. These positions have more in common with the poor postures we exhibit at a desk everyday than the athletic shapes we are seeking to develop.

Thankfully there are much smaller hurdles commercially available to enable junior athletes and smaller or less flexible athletes to perform the drills correctly. However if these are not available all is not lost. The drills can be performed just as well using 'imaginary hurdles'. This can actually have a great number of advantages. The hurdle will never be too high, it is free and it doesn't require stacking up afterwards. The only concession is that the athlete must be slightly more vigilant in pushing themselves to work to their fullest range on every step. Table 6.4 outlines some of the most effective hurdle drills, which are also discussed in chapter 11.

High-speed running
High-speed running, also known as strides, can essentially be thought of as practising running

fast. When we run fast many of the technical aspects of running that we have looked at start to fall into place naturally. The hips start to rise up, the chest lifts, the knees pick up and the foot contact moves from the heel fowards to the mid-foot. This gives the body an opportunity to experience how these positions feel and to coordinate them at high speed.

The most important point to remember when performing strides is they must be quicker than normal running but *always* below maximum sprint pace. It is crucial to hold something back in order to retain good control and stay relaxed. The distance should also be short, because fatigue will inevitably erode good technique. Typically a distance of 30–60 metres is ideal. Naturally the

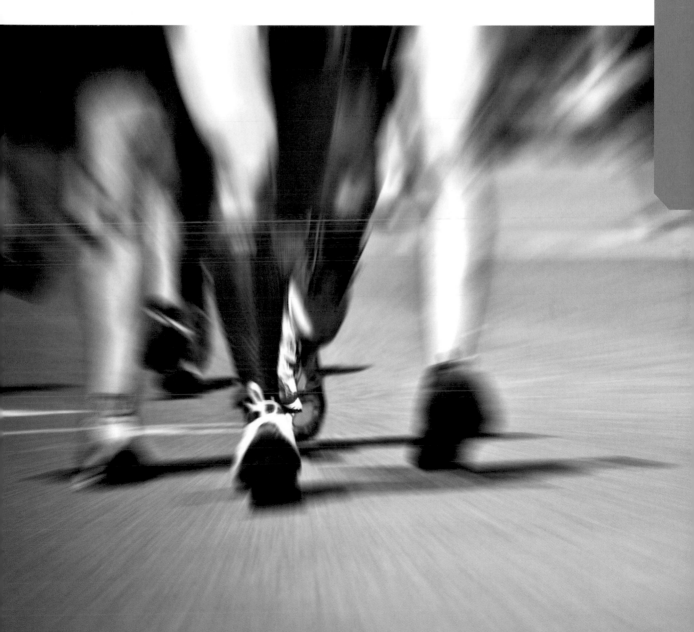

Table 6.4	Hurdle drills	
Drill	**Focus**	**Progressions**
Basic walk-through	Hip mobility, glute strength and global posture	Hold a light medicine ball above the head to increase the challenge to the posture
Reverse walk-through	Hip range and balance, glute strength	Step through two hurdles with second leg
Lateral skip	Opening the hips and ankle stiffness	
Down the side knee raise	Hip mobility	

distance can be extended in order to challenge the ability to maintain technique but we would suggest no more than 100 metres for technical strides.

One of the most effective ways of using strides is to alternate them with running drills. This provides an ideal opportunity to take the technical element of the drill and 'turn it into real running'. While there is no direct scientific evidence for it, it can also be useful to finish a heavy weights session with a few strides. One athlete described this as 'putting the running back in your legs'. In our experience this can be very helpful in avoiding a heavy legged feeling after a weights session.

Performance enhancement and power production

Finally we return to the place where we began at the start of the chapter – explosive-strength training and plyometrics to improve running performance.

Explosive-strength training

It is worth pointing out that explosive-strength training should be performed only if a good volume of basic strength work has been performed to underpin it. Strength through the various movement patterns will be required for good technique to be held when moving weights rapidly. It is also important to develop strength first as power is a product of both force and velocity. It is far easier to improve our capacity to produce force than our velocity and so this represents the most potent route to performance enhancement. We should always remember that a weak athlete can never be powerful. Many of the issues around developing lower body strength and power are covered in chapter 5. The programming of strength work is also covered in detail in chapter 8.

Plyometrics

Plyometrics is a form of exercise which has not previously featured in our discussion around training for the swim and the bike. This is because plyometrics is primarily concerned with stressing and developing the stretch shortening cycle to improve elastic or reactive strength. This plays a relatively minor role in the cyclical swim and cycle disciplines but, as we have seen, is fundamental to efficient and effective running performance.

Plyometrics originated in the former Soviet Union in the 1960s and was largely used by explosive track and field athletes. Plyometric exercises are typically made up of jumping-type activities with an emphasis on the rebound. Unfortunately many coaches become carried away with the 'sexier' exercises in this category and throw their athletes into highly demanding and technical jumps which they are not able to handle. This is not only dangerous but it is also unnecessary.

As we saw when discussing the fundamental principles of training we need to achieve overload (*see* chapter 1). This means that we must stress a physical quality to a greater extent than we are generally exposed to. For a sprinter or triple jumper that means that high-intensity plyometrics are needed to overload the athlete who experiences high forces as a fundamental part of their event. However for the endurance athlete it is a far simpler task to achieve stretch shortening cycle overload. What is the simplest method? Well how about running faster than race pace? Performing short sprints or speed efforts will put greater forces through the tendons, require quicker contact times and greater joint stiffness (*see* section 6.2). These are all the ideal ingredients of a plyometric exercise. On top of that it is also possible to use the work as technical running practice, the nervous system develops its ability to move the body quickly and if the session is structured correctly metabolic fitness gains can be achieved too! Consequently the number one choice of plyometric exercise for triathletes should clearly be sprinting.

In a similar fashion, faster running drills and skipping will also require a quicker ground contact than a typical running session and so these are also an efficient way of subtly including plyometric work in a training programme.

The more traditional plyometric exercises based on jumps are less specific but offer the benefit of developing muscular power effectively. The best example of these is the simple counter-movement jump (a brief dip followed by a rapid jump). This can be done in several ways including a jump on the spot, jump to a box and a straight-legged jump to a box. These alone will give good variety and allow the athlete to develop explosive power and coordination. Finally hopping exercises move one step closer to running specificity as they are performed on a single leg. This means that power must be produced while having the postural strength to keep the hips, knees and ankles stable.

There are many more plyometric exercises that could potentially be utilised by triathletes. However in general the technical demands of these exercises mean that a great deal of time is required to master the movement to make it both safe and effective. Given that there are simpler choices that are equally or more effective we would suggest that the precious training time of a triathlete can be more effectively spent elsewhere.

6.4 Summary

The running based component of the S&C programme must begin with an evaluation of where the limiting factor in the athlete's running lies. The most fruitful path will generally be in first developing the physical qualities to underpin good form, such as mobility and posture. As these qualities are developed they can start to be moulded into technical changes. Finally strength, power and reactive strength can be developed to boost the potency of good technique.

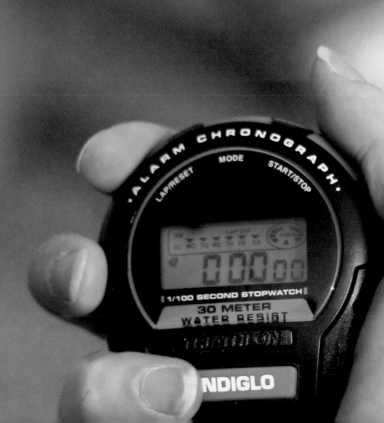

part 3

planning and programming

007
periodisation

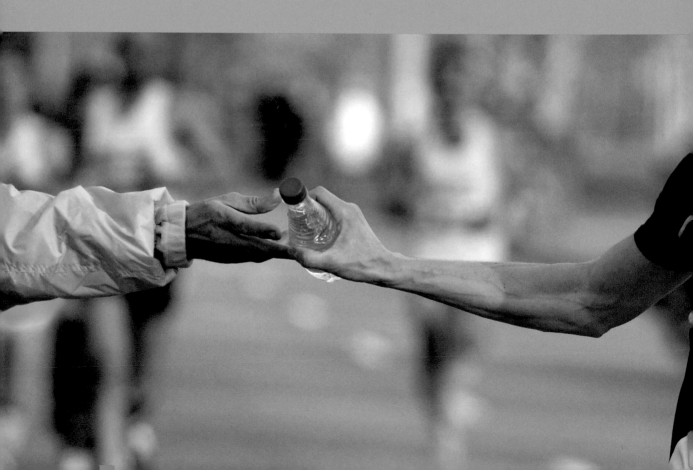

7.1 Introduction

Periodisation is a topic that is talked about a lot, but understood rarely. The concept originated from a Russian sports scientist named Matveyev in the 1960s. Since then Matveyev's ideas have been translated into English, adapted to fit many sports and widely reproduced. Unfortunately this processing and interpretation of the original ideas have led to much confusion and misunderstanding. In order to overcome much of the misinformation which has been published in books, magazines and the internet, it is necessary to strip the idea of periodisation to its core principles. Essentially periodisation is about the structured planning and progression of training. This can be done in a simplistic way or with great complexity. Fundamentally though if this structure and planning are not present then all other elements of the programme become meaningless, because the progress is doomed to slow to a stop and training will become stagnant.

As much as these statements may seem uncontroversial and almost obvious it is staggering how many triathletes fall into this trap. Athletes find a collection of exercises that they like and feel like they are doing some good. These get put together to form a session that is then repeated week by week, month by month and eventually year by year. It is for this reason that periodisation is one of the biggest differences between training or simply exercising. Both are equally hard work, but one leads somewhere whereas the other just feels good at the time.

There is no way even the most dedicated athlete can hope to train effectively all of their physical qualities to their full potential throughout the entire season. By evaluating how training emphasis, volumes and intensity will change throughout the season a broad and thorough programme can be designed. Finally as you approach the key event of the season the taper of the training programme becomes critical. Take your foot off the gas too much and hard work through the season will be wasted. Fail to taper sufficiently and you'll lack the sharpness to hit your true potential.

Of course all of these principles of periodisation should already be in place in a triathlete's wider training programme. Therefore we will concern ourselves with outlining some of the basic concepts of periodisation in general and then look at how they apply specifically to the strength and conditioning programme.

7.2 Basic concepts in periodisation

The first aspect of periodisation that must be addressed is the division of the calendar into phases of training. This provides a background and a framework for manipulation of training. Training is broken down into phases or cycles and is done on three levels; micro-, meso- and macrocycles.

Microcycles

The shortest phases of training are the microcycles, which are typically one week in duration. Some coaches do not like to be restricted by seven-day cycles and move away from this traditional set-up. Theoretically this is great as it shows imagination and means that training modes can be alternated in ways that work best for the athlete rather than having to fit into a recurrent seven-day cycle. However in real life this is often highly impractical, particularly for those without the luxury of being full-time athletes. Most of us need the regular routine of knowing that we will run on a Monday, swim with the club on a Tuesday, etc. The problems of changing this on a weekly basis are likely to far outweigh the benefits. The microcycle gives us the basic set-up for how our sessions fit together and what we will be doing. The specific volumes and intensities can then be manipulated through the mesocycle.

Mesocycles

The mesocycle is the tool that allows us to shift the emphasis of training throughout the year. If this is done correctly then each cycle will build on the gains made in the previous. The classic example of this is when a strength block is followed by a power block to allow the body to express gains in force explosively. Most commonly the mesocycle will last 4–6 weeks. The logic behind this is that these durations allow enough time for physical adaptation to occur but also give an opportunity for rest. For example, a four-week cycle may build over three weeks with the fourth week being a recovery week. This is a perfectly logical system – provided the athlete is working at a level sufficiently advanced to stress them physically and justify the use of recovery weeks. The importance of technique and movement control means that novices to S&C will be largely limited by their technical ability rather than physical capacity during the early stages of training. Sadly many coaches and athletes fail to recognise this and

restrict themselves to the rigid models presented in many text books. Ultimately though there is no law stating that a block must end after six weeks! If progress is still being made and the competition calendar allows, there is no reason why a block cannot be extended significantly beyond this.

Macrocycles

Finally we have the macrocycle. In general this refers to the overall picture of the year and will conclude with a competitive period through the summer. More advanced athletes may aim for a double peak with a targeted competition early in the year (perhaps a sprint event) followed by a rebuilding towards a second key event later in the year. Those with several years of experience and taking a very focused approach to their sport may plan macrocycles to build over several years with a different technical focus each year. The classic example of this is the Olympic athlete who may plan over a four-year period towards an Olympic games.

Table 7.1 gives a very basic example of how a periodised plan may be mapped out. The volume row illustrates how the amount of work performed each week will cycle. The emphasis of each block shows each mesocycle building on the previous.

Table 7.1	Sample periodised planner											
Week commencing	3 Oct.	10 Oct.	17 Oct.	24 Oct.	31 Oct.	7 Nov.	14 Nov.	21 Nov.	28 Nov.	5 Dec.	12 Dec.	19 Dec.
Week no.	1	2	3	4	5	6	7	8	9	10	11	12
Volume	L	M	H	R	L	M	H	R	L	M	H	R
Block	1				2				3			
Emphasis	Conditioning				General strength				Maximum strength			

Note: L – light, M – medium, H – heavy, R – recovery

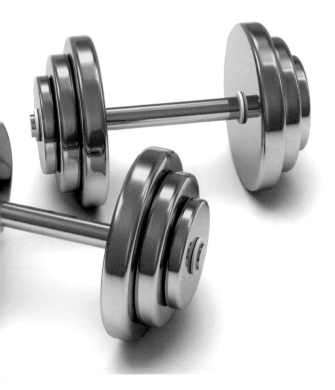

transfers most closely to our event. Some people get so seduced by this type of work and its apparent specificity that they struggle to move away from it at any time of year. However if we start on this type of work in October, where can we take the programme from here? We either face inevitable plateaux very early in the year or must move towards less specific work just as we need the transfer most!

By starting with general work and moving to specific, each time a plateau looms the emphasis is shifted slightly and the body can make fresh adaptations. Also this logical development of 'building blocks' makes the final stages of training more effective. As we have already learned, a weak athlete cannot benefit from power training, and sprint training will be a blunt tool if technique and control are poor, etc. Therefore by putting the correct sequence of blocks together the end result can be much greater than the sum of the parts.

7.3 Periodisation models

There are a huge number of periodisation models in circulation, each with various strengths and weaknesses. It is important to bear in mind that S&C will represent only one of four elements of training for the triathlete and so a hugely complex periodisation model is not warranted. Therefore we will simply look at a few of the most common methods. The biggest debate revolves around so-called linear versus non-linear (also known as undulating) models.

Linear periodisation

The linear model is the most commonly discussed and sees a number of general patterns develop throughout the training year, which gradually shifts throughout the season from general to specific. Naturally we want our training around competition time to be work that relates and

As the season progresses there is also an overarching shift from high volume to high intensity. Through the winter, well away from competition, there is no risk in accumulating fatigue. Of course this must be managed effectively so that sufficient recovery is put in place to allow for adaptation and super-compensation (*see* chapter 1). However through these months the athlete has their best opportunity to accumulate large amounts of work. Because this volume is high the intensity is relatively low. This is a natural balance as at the start of the season strength levels will generally be low and so the capacity for true high-intensity work is limited. (Care must be taken not to confuse total effort with intensity, because high-volume sessions will always feel hard). As the season develops and competition approaches the need for freshness becomes more apparent. Therefore there is a natural drop-off in volume of S&C work. At this stage we should be seeking to do small amounts of very high-quality work. This allows us to peak for performance by minimising fatigue and maximising strength qualities.

Non-linear periodisation

The biggest difference in the non-linear model is the manipulation of volume and intensity on a daily basis. Rather than having a steady progression across weeks and months, the undulating model shifts from day to day. This is particularly important for more advanced athletes. If an athlete is performing several heavy strength sessions per week and has a good strength base, this sophisticated variance of training is important to avoid burnout and to maintain progression. However the vast majority of triathletes are unlikely to perform more than two sessions per week, and one of these is likely to be more movement and technique based. In this situation a basic linear model is most appropriate.

Conjugate model

The conjugate model is a form of non-linear periodisation which is based on the theory that all strength qualities may be developed simultaneously. Each block may have a specific focus whereby one quality is stressed preferentially, but this does not mean that other qualities are ignored entirely. This makes a lot of sense for a number of reasons. Following a progression of qualities through the year means that only a relatively small percentage of the training year is spent focused on the key goal. For example, in seeking to become more powerful many athletes will follow a programme that trains power for only two months of the whole year. For the same reason there will only be one point in the calendar when these qualities have come to the

fore. For athletes who wish to compete at a good level throughout a long season this is clearly far from ideal.

This all sounds too good to be true though – you can train everything all of the time and improve all strength qualities simultaneously! There are potential pitfalls though. If the programme is not skilfully put together it will end up not being periodised at all, as the emphasis remains the same from block-to-block. Similarly the opportunity to overload a specific strength quality is limited in comparison with the classic model. If there is one quality that is a limiting factor to performance it may be more desirable to focus on this and make maximal gains rather than trying to achieve too much elsewhere.

Which model works best for me?

The answer very much depends of the individual. We would recommend that the novice strength trainer coming into an S&C programme in an organised way for the first time loosely follows a linear model. This will enable them to focus on developing a solid foundation of technique and basic/general strength in a steady and targeted way.

Assuming that this first season has been successful in terms of establishing a good base of strength, conditioning and technique it may be wise to start to move towards a conjugate type system. As this second year will be more focused on performance we want to make sure we spend as much time as possible developing our speed and power. This may still develop along the theme of a linear year but with a few other elements thrown into each block. As the years go by this shifting closer and closer to the conjugate system is probably appropriate as the level of strength training maturity increases.

Of course this is a personal view (albeit based on years of experience with athletes). Many will still swear by the classic models and will stick to this unswervingly year in, year out. Ultimately the question needs to be asked – am I still getting better? If the answer is yes then no theoretical argument can trump the evidence seen in the gym.

7.4 Misunderstandings and common errors in periodisation

As much as it is important to give guidance as to how to periodise a programme, it is almost equally important to state what not to do. There is a lot of poorly interpreted information available on the subject, and many models are put forward that are not suitable for triathlon. Therefore we can save a lot of wasted time by looking at some of the most common mistakes and problems.

The dominance of American literature

Although modern periodisation is a concept that came from Russia, much of the interpretation of this work and the popular texts come from the USA. One of the factors that stands out in US sports is the importance of size and bulk. As a result most of these models tend to have a hypertrophy (muscle building) phase at the start of the season. Clearly this is not suitable for triathletes looking to maximise power-to-weight ratio. Because these sports also require maximum strength and high-load power, these are also the end goals of many periodised plans. As a result technical ability, reactive strength and body control work tend to be somewhat overlooked within the calendar.

These text books do not need to be ignored completely, but following them to the letter will lead to inevitable problems. When reading any of these books or websites it is critical to bear in mind that some of the fundamental concepts can be powerful but the specifics may need adapting.

Overemphasising the theme of the block

Even when using a linear model of periodisation, several strength qualities can and should still be developed within the same session. Because we tend to talk in basic terms such as a 'strength block' or a 'power block' this is sometimes interpreted to mean that only exercises that develop these qualities should be included. This is always an error that will yield poor results. Imagine an athlete who followed this path and

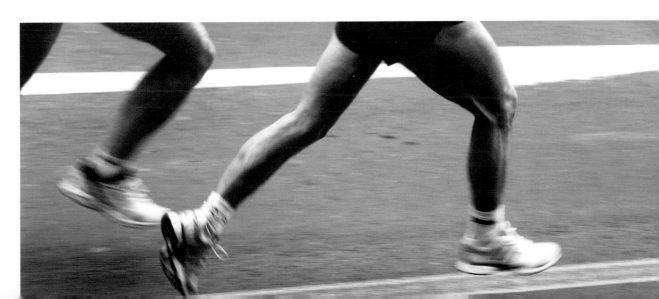

trained using four-week blocks in strength, power and speed. By the end of the speed block they would not have trained strength for two months! It should be obvious that the benefit of four weeks of training will easily be lost entirely if ignored for eight weeks. The amount of work required to maintain this quality is far less than that required to build it, but there must be some maintenance work – or detraining is inevitable.

Failing to stick to the plan

The subtle shifts in intensity that occur through each micro- and mesocycle are fundamental for making progress in performances. Anyone can train hard, but training smart is far more rare. Far too often I have seen athletes turn up for a planned hard session feeling a little tired. Sometimes we need to back off, although there are also times to push through. These athletes inevitably take the session down a notch, and a hard session becomes a moderate session. These same athletes also like the feeling of having done a session that felt like 'good training'. As a result planned light sessions, which allow for recovery, end up being pushed on to become moderate. The pattern for these athletes becomes clear when you step back, as there is hardly any variation in their training intensity or volume. This can only lead to stagnation and a failure to make further gains.

Sticking to the plan too closely

At the risk of completely contradicting the previous point, it is a huge mistake to treat the periodised plan as being perfect and written in stone. Imagine the following scenario: an athlete has planned to move from light to moderate then heavy intensities of a course in three progressive strength training weeks. During week 2 she feels really strong and wants to lift heavy but holds back as the plan says it is a moderate week. The following week she comes to the gym feeling flat

and fails to lift her target weights. This is a classic case of sticking to the plan too closely. Our bodies do not adapt in a nice, tidy linear fashion as a plan may require. While we can start to anticipate better how we will respond through experience of training over time these changes can never be fully anticipated by the plan. This is partly just the way we are made and partly down to other factors in daily life, which all influence how we feel. Therefore it is vital that we keep licence to push on when we are firing on all cylinders and drop the pace off when it just isn't there.

7.5 Tapering and peaking for performance

Each phase of training is important in its own right. However as with racing itself it's not how you start but how you finish that counts. Many a good S&C plan has been ruined by a failure to get the run-in to the event itself correct. While it is a mistake to fail to back off from training as competitions approach this is more commonly seen in the 'fitness' element of a triathlete's training programme. When it comes to S&C the reverse is often the case. After dedicatedly building strength qualities through the preparation period the athlete frequently discards this element of their training entirely with several weeks of training to go. For the S&C coach this is hugely frustrating as hard-earned gains are lost to detraining and are never let loose on competition.

These days the science of the taper has been refined to a precisely engineered process. Much of this is thanks to a researcher by the name of Dr Inigo Mujika. His work has taught us that there is more to the taper than simply reducing fatigue to leave the athlete fresh for competition. When performed correctly a well-planned taper can actually enhance performance beyond the removal

Table 7.2	Effects of volume reduction on performance
Decrease in volume (per cent)	**Effects**
≤20	No change
21–40	Small change
41–60	Biggest positive change
≥61	Some positive change but risk of detraining

Source: Tapering & Peaking for Optimal Performance, Mujika, I., Human Kinetics, 2009

of fatigue. So what does a perfect taper look like? Although it is a very individual process that requires a certain amount of experimentation, Dr Mujika has identified certain factors that are consistently seen in the best tapers.

How does training change during the taper?

The number one rule is that the taper should mean a reduction of volume *not* intensity. This means that we are still practising high-quality work and staying sharp, but the reduced volume allows the body to recover much more quickly than in a normal session. During normal training the aim is deliberately to induce the cycle of damage-repair known as supercompensation. This is the basis of all training (*see* chapter 1). However this is not the goal of a taper session. Here we are simply aiming to 'keep in touch' with our strength and power. In fact many athletes utilise so-called 'activation sessions' very close to competition (24 hours or less) in order to feel really sharp.

How much should I reduce volume by?

The reduction in volume should ideally be 40–60 per cent. The effects of different levels of reduction in volume are described in table 7.2. The actual reduction will depend on many individual factors, including how much S&C work we have started with. There is also a degree of personal preference and just what works. However studies have consistently shown that dropping volume below 40 per cent or failing to drop to at least 80 per cent will yield inferior results

How far out from competition should the taper begin?

Dr Mujika recommends a taper duration of 2–6 weeks as optimal. The amount and significance of your S&C will influence this.

7.6 Summary

The key to periodising your training effectively is to begin with an established process based on sound principles. By engaging in this process and slowly refining small details it is possible to get an excellent insight as to how the body responds and adjust the model accordingly. Therefore initial plans are based on theory and over the years they become based more on experience of what works. This plan will also change over time as the athlete develops. Remember what worked in year one may not work in year two. Similarly just because a particular plan is in a book or another triathlete has had success with one does not make their plan the best one for you.

008
putting it all together

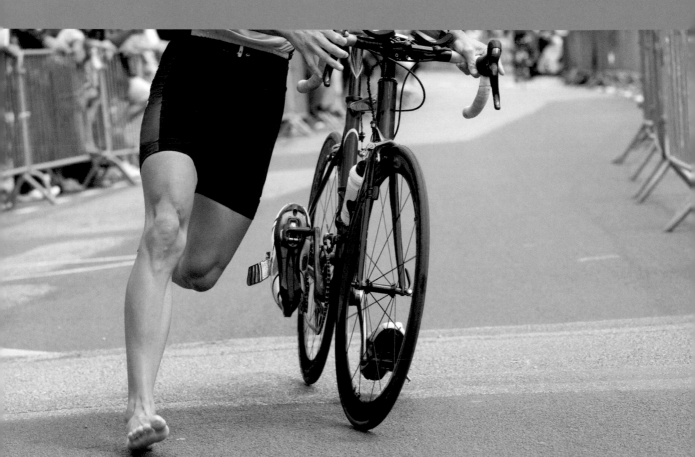

8.1 Introduction

Now that we have reviewed all the evidence supporting strength and conditioning and the methods available we come to one final but critical aspect – the art of putting it all into practice. There are many learned sports scientists and well-read triathletes who fall at the final hurdle when it comes to planning their sessions. A fully rounded S&C programme is like a great recipe – there are lots of ingredients and how you put them together is crucial to how it ends up. In chapter 1 we discussed some of the founding principles of training such as overload, progression and specificity. Now we can look at some of the key components in the practice of strength and conditioning training.

8.2 Measuring what you do

In order to achieve the aforementioned principles of training with any level of precision it is vital that we are able to measure what we do. This is generally defined separately by volume (amount of work) and intensity (difficulty of work). Each time an exercise is performed this is known as a repetition (rep), a group of these is described as a set. During general weight training, volume is typically measured and organised through the sets and reps system. An athlete may for example perform 3 sets of 10 reps (3 x 10). Sprints and drills are easily measured by the distance covered, e.g. 5 x 30m.

In the vast majority of programmes this system works perfectly well. However there are times when this way of thinking may be somewhat restrictive. Conditioning exercises are sometimes better measured by time rather than repetitions. Of course this is the only option with isometric exercises such as the plank, where there can be only one repetition (or even zero as there is no

movement). As we will discover later, in some forms of training the amount of time under tension is as important as the number of movements. For these exercises a set of 10 performed quickly may take the same amount of time as a set of five performed slowly. Therefore some may argue that measuring TUT (time under tension) is a more accurate way of measuring work in some cases.

The monitoring of intensity can be a slightly more complex affair. Traditional gym training generally uses the load lifted to monitor intensity. Some will simply record the weight moved, whereas others note the percentage of the athletes 1RM (one-repetition maximum lift). This is generally reserved for high-level strength training though and is unlikely to be suitable for triathletes. Part of the reason for this is that most of our exercises will be focused on developing control and good-quality movement. Therefore these are generally not appropriate to perform with extremely heavy weights. The per cent rep max method also requires regular testing on each exercise, which can be highly impractical. There are many other problems that can complicate the task of measuring intensity: for example, 50kg may be very easy for an athlete to lift in a double-legged squat performed in October, but very heavy in a single-leg squat in November. However if we just record the amount lifted times the reps and sets this may look as if the two months were the same intensity! We can also add in the complication of bodyweight exercises such as press-ups. As the feet are in contact with the ground the whole body weight is not being lifted, but how do we know how much is?

These are just some of a huge number of issues that S&C coaches wrestle with when monitoring the intensity of strength training. The thing to remember as a triathlete is that S&C is just one component of your training. We also need to

Table 8.1	Sample gym training diary				
Name: *James Barnes*			Session Date: *12 Jan. 2012*		
Exercise	Comments	Sets	Reps	Weight	
single-leg squats	*Knees were wobbling a bit*	*4*	*8*	*30kg*	
Press-ups	*Felt strong, increase next week*	*3*	*12*	*n/a*	
side plank	*Hard work*	*3*	*35s*	*n/a*	

achieve just one simple but crucial goal through our monitoring – to be able to see if we are getting better and to be able to plan our sessions with precision. Therefore I would strongly urge the use of the simplest system possible to record the volume and intensity so that it is possible to judge whether more or less on any given exercise has been done. The best way to do this is through a very simple training diary such as in table 8.1.

8.3 Designing the session

As we start to put pen to paper a number of questions will (hopefully) arise as to exactly how the session should look and what are the reasons behind it. This is an important point as by understanding exactly why a session looks as it does will enable the athlete to judge if it is the most effective way of doing things.

How many reps should I do for power exercises?

So, we know that we are going to measure our exercises using the set–rep system, but how do we decide how many sets and reps to perform of each exercise? Contrary to standard gym culture and the

popular prescription of exercise by physiotherapists the answer is not always 3 sets of 10! In fact these variables are extremely important in determining the outcome of the exercise, so they warrant good consideration. Figure 8.1 is a guide to the appropriate number of repetitions for a given goal.

Of course these goals will come to fruition only if the intensity is high enough. Just performing 1–5 reps of a very light weight will clearly not make you stronger! Working in these rep ranges is generally more suitable for experienced weight trainers, who have the capacity to challenge themselves in just a few repetitions. Most novices will find that the best weight they can perform safely for five reps they can actually do for several more (therefore the load is too light). Alternatively if they use a weight that they can perform for only a few reps their technique will break down and the lift becomes poor quality and dangerous.

If technique and control do not allow for heavier sets then the goal of training becomes slightly different and the programming changes accordingly. Here we are focused on motor patterning and basic control and may use a lighter

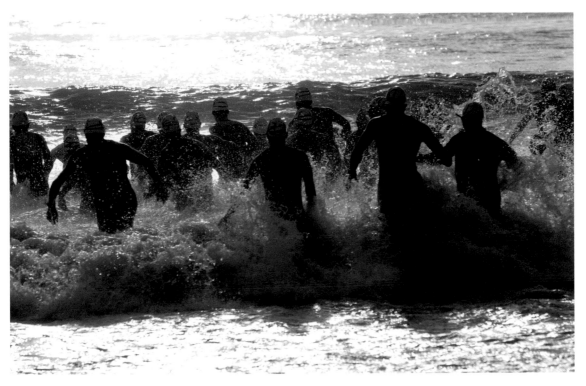

Max strength
• 1–5 reps per set
• 15–25 reps total

Power
• 2–5 reps per set
• 15–30 reps total

Strength endurance
• 5–8 reps per set
• 20–35 reps total

Motor patterning/hypertrophy
• 8–12 reps
• 20–35 reps total

Conditioning
• 30–90 seconds per set

Figure 8.1 Repetition guideline

weight for 8–12 repetitions. The reason for this number is simply that is provides more chances to practise the movement than the lower rep ranges. Theoretically this could be increased further but this leads to fatigue, and technique is likely to break down. This is not desirable in the early stages, and each set should be finished fresh enough that the technique is still as good as the first repetition. For this reason there is nothing wrong with breaking the session down into a larger number of sets of fewer reps (e.g. 6 x 5 rather than 3 x 10). This allows the athlete to remain fresh and also provides more opportunity for a coach to give feedback. Once the technique has been drilled the numbers can then increase so that it can be performed repeatedly well.

The 8–12 rep range is also described as being appropriate for hypertrophy (muscle building). This often causes a lot of confusion and fear in

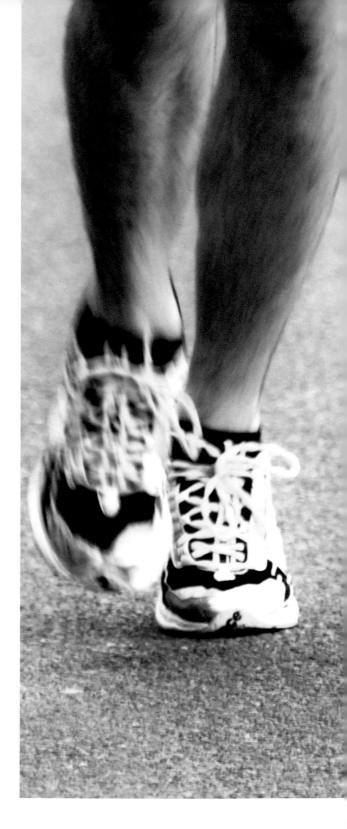

athletes who are keen to avoid 'bulking up'. Thankfully though these fears are unfounded. While the number of repetitions may be similar to a bodybuilding-type programme there are many other factors that differ. These include the way in which the session is structured (*see* below), rest between sets, nutrition and genetics. The typical triathlete with lots of slow-twitch muscle fibres and a high volume of endurance training is in no danger whatsoever of becoming too big.

When it comes to developing power (which is generally a key end goal in almost any S&C programme), the number of repetitions performed is very important. What is the one thing that differentiates a power movement from all other aspects of strength? Speed. If we try to perform a large number of repetitions in one set we will inevitably become fatigued. The first victim of fatigue is speed. It is for this reason that the guideline of 2–5 repetitions for power exercises should be pretty well adhered to.

How many conditioning sets should I do?

Finally we come to conditioning. Here we have chosen to look at the time spent working rather than a fixed number of repetitions. As we have touched on already, the goal of conditioning is essentially to increase the work tolerance of the muscle and allow it to be able to perform for longer. Because of the variability of repetition speed it is more useful to focus on time than the number of repetitions. This also allows the athlete to place greater focus on technique and maintain form rather than becoming ragged in an attempt to produce an enormous number of repetitions.

To some extent the number of sets is determined by the number of reps. A good guideline is to perform 20–35 repetitions per exercise. A heavy strength session may use 5 sets of 5 (25 total reps), whereas a motor patterning exercise may be based on 4 sets of 8 (32 reps). These numbers are by no means set in stone and should just be considered a guideline.

How long should I rest between sets?

This is one of the most important yet overlooked aspects of training. A brilliantly designed session can be entirely ruined if the rest between sets is wrong. The issue ultimately comes down to whether or not accumulated fatigue is desirable or disastrous. We have already seen that fatigue will ruin power development. It will also compromise technique when developing movement pattern. Therefore the rest between sets for both these goals should be sufficient that each set is performed as well as the first. A good guide to this is somewhere in the region of two minutes (there are ways of making training more efficient though without compromising on quality – this is known as training density). The same guidelines apply to strength training. As we saw in chapter 1, many of the adaptations to strength training occur in the nervous system. For these to be effective it is important that the quality remains high throughout.

When it comes to conditioning though it is essential that fatigue accumulates though the sets. Our primary goal is to induce as much fatigue in the muscle as possible in order that we will be able to perform for longer next time. Therefore rest should be kept to a minimum (20–45 seconds). Often rest can be kept to zero by performing a series of exercises in quick succession (see below). For those interested in gaining muscle mass, the rest should also be kept to 45–90 seconds between sets. In this way the final set should be extremely hard work with failure coming around the last rep.

How many times should I train each week?

The number of sessions per week is another aspect of S&C which, if a little imagination is used, can have a dramatic impact on the amount that can be achieved. Typically triathletes will use 1–2 sessions per week, both of which will be 45–60 minutes long and circuit based. We have already seen how the circuit obsession can be hugely limiting, but it could be argued that the fixation with one-hour sessions is equally problematic. By dividing strength and conditioning into targeted mini-sessions it is possible to be both more effective and more efficient.

I would generally recommend that two sessions per week is ideal for strength work. One session may be acceptable for maintenance (if you are maintaining relatively low levels of strength) but with a full seven days between sessions it is very difficult for all but the weakest of athletes to move forwards. There may be some merit in three sessions per week, and indeed this can be highly effective during intensive blocks where strength training is a primary focus. However the time and training constraints of three sessions generally make this impractical on a long-term continuous basis for most of us.

Conditioning work, especially rehab, can and often should be performed more than twice a week. Immediately this highlights the problem of putting all of our S&C together in one session. A small routine can be devised that can either be performed at home or be combined with other training sessions.

Finally we come to drills and special strength work. Clearly it is highly impractical trying to combine these with a traditional gym session. What's more, using technical practice is an excellent method of

Strength and Conditioning for Triathlon

warm-up as it not only makes use of dead time and junk kilometres, but is ideal preparation for the forthcoming session as good technique is drilled to 'prime' for the forthcoming session.

How fast should the exercises be performed?

Most exercises should be done at a good steady tempo. The typical athlete will perform lifts too quickly in an attempt to finish the set more quickly or to enable them to lift a heavier weight. As a general guideline a tempo of two seconds on the effort (concentric phase) and three seconds on the return (eccentric phase) will allow for a good quality of technique. For example, a squat would be performed three seconds on the way down and two seconds on the way up. Often this eccentric phase (which is of great value) is rushed and the athlete never has full control. Moving the weight

too quickly means that we fail to train the whole movement as momentum takes over. Many an athlete would improve their sessions greatly if they simply forgot about the number on the bar and moved more slowly.

Of course moving slowly is not conducive to developing power. Therefore any exercise aimed at improving power should be performed as explosively as possible (without losing control or technique). This is often something that doesn't come naturally to the endurance athlete who spends hours every week training the nervous system to perform submaximal efforts repeatedly. The experienced strength-trained athlete will be able to summon the ability to produce a single effort of huge power in an instant. Therefore mental preparation and focus are critical for the triathlete to develop this ability. You should

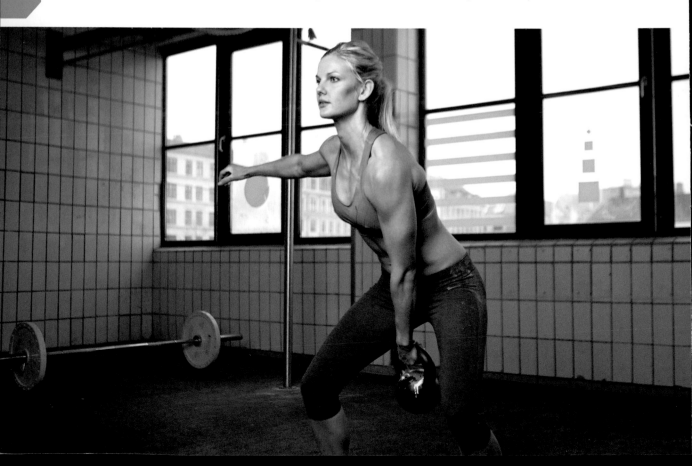

practise taking at least 30 seconds before each set to focus on what you are going to do and really dig deep to produce everything you have in an instant.

Once again though nothing is set in stone and there is always plenty of room for creativity and imagination in the gym (just as long as it is backed up by sensible scientific principles). Just try a set of 6 x 10-second press-ups (one rep lasts five seconds down and five seconds up) and the athlete will see there are many ways of mixing things up.

In what order should the exercises be performed?

Few triathletes will not have heard of the circuit session. This, for the rare few who have not tried a circuit, consists of a session whereby exercises are performed one after another for a single set with little or no rest. Typically the circuit will contain 8–10 exercises, and the athlete will go around the circuit three times. The reason these are so popular with triathletes is that they are regarded as strength–endurance training. There is logic to this and indeed there is some value to the session. However they also represent the classic inability to step away briefly from endurance and develop a broader spectrum of strength qualities and movement skills.

Using circuits exclusively is a very limited approach, but they can still be utilised effectively in conjunction with other ways of organising training. A more balanced approach sees strength and power exercises, which demand quality and concentration, performed at the start of the session. These can then be followed by mini-circuits that may focus on a specific area, such as a trunk conditioning circuit, or a foot and ankle circuit. As we have learned, the strength and power exercises require a reasonable recovery

between sets. This sits uncomfortably with some triathletes who want to feel as if they are constantly working. It can also seem somewhat inefficient, which doesn't sit well with busy training schedules. The best way to get around this is to increase training density through the use of super-sets. This means combining two exercises, which are performed in succession followed by a rest. In order to prevent a negative effect on the main exercise, the second movement should be one that will not impact on it. A great way of doing this is to combine a strength exercise with a prehab exercise: for example, single-leg squats may be paired with the hop-stick exercise. This not only helps to keep the session moving but also provides an efficient way of getting lower-level exercise done without dragging the session out excessively.

It is important not to become too rigid when planning sessions. However figure 8.2 shows one way to structure a session. Movement preparation includes stretching and mobility work, which serves as preparation for the main session and helps to 'set the body up' for the work ahead. Technique and motor patterning work should be performed when fresh. This also gives an opportunity to practise techniques prior to the demanding and intense strength and power work. The session can then be concluded with the hard conditioning exercises, safe in the knowledge that nothing needs to be left in the tank.

Figure 8.2 Suggested session structure

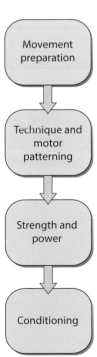

8.4 Determining training focus

One of the great joys of a multi-event sport is the fact that there are so many different elements of training. Not only are there three times as many disciplines within the sport than most activities, but each of these can also be further divided into technical, tactical, endurance, speed, strength, etc. While this adds to the variety and enjoyment of training it can also be somewhat daunting for the uninitiated when planning a training programme. The same can be said for embarking on a S&C programme to improve triathlon performance.

A number of questions are likely to arise, such as how much time to devote to S&C, how important is it for me and what should my focus be? Perhaps the best approach is to deal with these three important questions in reverse order. Once you have identified the areas that you will focus on it is much easier to decide the significance of this within the overall training programme. Training priorities can be thought of on several levels (*see* figure 8.3). It should be noted that special strength refers to work that is directly performance related but still distinct from the sport, whereas specific strength is very highly related (*see* chapter 11)

It is important to realise that most athletes will be working on multiple levels at any one time (although almost never on all levels). An athlete new to S&C will generally begin working on levels 1 and 2. More experienced athletes are likely to start the season on levels 1 and 2 and gradually shift towards levels 2 and 3 as the season progresses. Only for a very brief period will the most advanced trainers focus on levels 3 and 4. It is important to remember that the athlete is describing their training status in terms of S&C rather than as a triathlete. There are many experienced elite triathletes who can be considered only novice in terms of S&C. This process requires the athlete to evaluate their current performance. There are a few key questions that may help direct them and clarify how S&C will impact on their season.

How much does injury impact on the quality and quantity of an athlete's training?

If injury, or the fear of injury, is causing a loss of training time or causing sessions to be changed then this alone is justification for a significant focus to be placed on rehab/prehab. Ironically by sacrificing triathlon training for S&C the ability to train for longer and not miss sessions can be increased through improved mechanics and tissue tolerance.

How much progression is the athlete making in each of the three disciplines and what are the limiting factors?

It is a natural part of training that, as time goes by, gains begin to plateau. This will be the case for many triathletes reading this text. This is not

Level 4
• Specific strength

Level 3
• Max strength & power (special strength)

Level 2
• Base strength (capacity & control), tissue conditioning

Level 1
• Rehabilitation & movement dysfunction, gym techniques

Figure 8.3 Priority of training focus

to say that gains are not still being made but they are much slower. The common response to this is to try to find more opportunities to train for longer, to squeeze in an extra session, etc. As a result the idea of actually *dropping* a session to make way for S&C is completely counterintuitive and quite scary. Rest assured though this is the perfect time to train smarter and kick the performance on again.

Those who are entirely new to the sport may feel that their time is best spent 'learning the trade' and just building a good volume of swimming, cycling and running. This is entirely logical and almost certainly the best path to making initial gains. However it is still prudent to include an element of S&C within the programme. By improving conditioning and movement quality the athlete will be better equipped to develop their sports skills and will greatly reduce the likelihood of sustaining an overuse injury further down the line. The significance of this will of course depend on how well the athlete moves and their starting predisposition to injury. For some one session per week can be viewed as prudent insurance, whereas for others several sessions will be required in order to be able to train.

How much emphasis does an athlete place on each discipline?

A great part of having an athletic development focus to training (i.e., developing athletic qualities, which underpin all sports performance) is that the multi-eventer does not require a separate session for each discipline. The squats that they perform to strengthen the trunk for swimming also build strength in the legs for cycling and improve hip mobility for running! Therefore by addressing the athlete first and the sport second we become much more effective. This is particularly true in the early part of the season. As competition approaches,

training will naturally become more specific to each discipline, as special strength becomes more the focus (*see* chapter 7). However this work will also start to become part of general triathlon training rather than dedicated S&C sessions

8.5 Novel methods of training

As a coach who continually receives catalogues full of ever weirder and more wonderful toys I know better than most that there are literally hundreds of novelty training methods that gain popularity through health clubs and fitness magazines. These are often backed by a great deal of hype, which can make them seem quite compelling. While there is nothing wrong with these methods of training *per se* it is important that we critically evaluate what they bring to the programme before we introduce them. Always remember – there is very little that the athlete cannot achieve through their own body weight and a few rudimentary tools! However for the curious here are a few of the novel methods that may add some value when used at the right time.

Suspension training systems

These systems, such as those by TRX, are based on gymnastic rings and use the athlete's own body weight as a form of resistance. In order to increase or decrease the resistance the dynamics of the exercise can be changed to use more or less of the athlete's body weight. These exercises are excellent for athletic development, as good performance requires full control of the athlete's body – just as in sport. The systems are also highly portable, which can be useful for those who travel regularly or do not have access to a gym.

Overall these are an excellent training tool for triathletes. Perhaps the biggest limitation to the system is the inability to add additional load in the way in which dumb-bell and barbell exercises can.

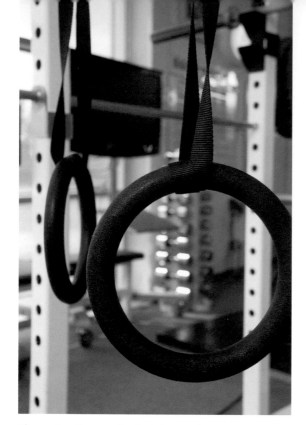

Figure 8.4 Suspension training system

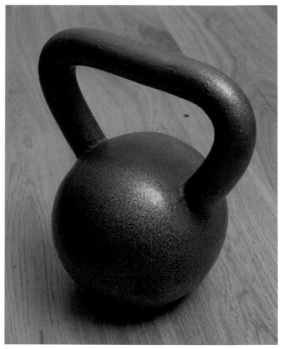

Figure 8.5 Kettlebells

Therefore these, as with all tools, are a great addition as part of a programme, but may be limited if viewed as the bulk or only element to a programme.

Kettlebells

Originating from Russia, the kettlebell is an incredibly simple tool, which is essentially a cast-iron ball with a handle. Kettlebells are most suitable for ballistic exercises such as swings and throws. The handle makes these challenges much more natural than with a dumb-bell. Despite the claims that this represents a complete training system, it is actually beneficial in only very specific tasks. Many of the overhead movements such as the kettlebell snatch combine power, trunk strength and shoulder stability. Therefore there are a number of exercises that can be used to assist elements of swim strength.

A note of caution – the kettlebell may be considered a Jack of all trades and a master of none. The practicality of holding the weight restricts large loads being used. Therefore it is far from the first port of call for power development. Similarly the ballistic nature of the exercises means control of shoulder stability may also be compromised.

Resistance bands

These are an ingenious method of overcoming one of the biggest weaknesses of traditional barbell exercises. All sports movements involve an acceleration through the movement, whereas gym exercises typically slow down as the end of range is reached. The mechanics of an exercise such as a squat also mean that, while the bottom of the movement is very hard, the final part is very easy. The use of resistance bands addresses both of

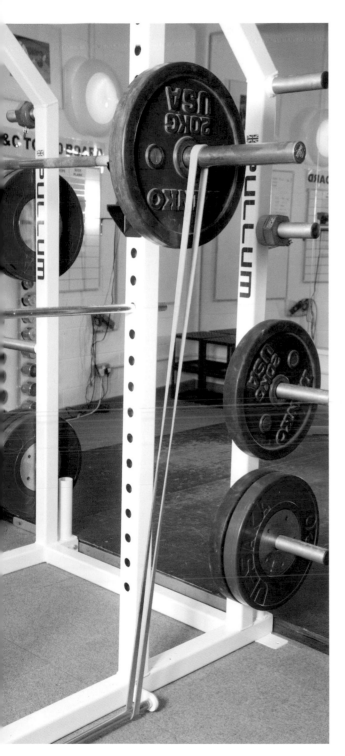

Figure 8.6 Resistance bands

these problems. The bands are attached either directly above or directly below the barbell and the bar itself. This then changes the dynamics of the exercise so that the load is increased toward the top of the movement. This causes the lifter to have to work hard throughout the range and reduces the natural urge to decelerate.

Theoretically these can be used by anyone at any stage. However they are best saved for times when ordinary barbell exercises have been mastered and gains have plateaued in order to give a fresh boost to training. Caution should also be used, as the bands take some getting used to and can easily end in embarrassment and landing in a heap!

8.6 Case studies

One of my inspirations for writing this book was the lack of helpful literature on the subject of S&C for triathlon. Too often I have read session plans that are recommended as being 'sessions to make you stronger' or 'the ultimate workout to improve your speed'. For me this goes against the very nature of good S&C, which focuses on the qualities of the individual first and foremost. As such it is impossible for this book to tell the athlete exactly what their session should contain. Instead my aim is to provide enough information on the science, theory and practice of strength training that the athlete can apply it to their own circumstance for maximum effect. However it is always useful to have some real-life examples to help lift the science off the page. Therefore the case studies below are highlighted to give some idea of how sessions may look in real life and also hopefully to fire the imagination to enable the athlete to use creative workouts to truly impact on their triathlon.

CASE STUDY THE ABSOLUTE BEGINNER

Andrew had been involved in triathlon for just over two years during which time he had been completely bitten by the triathlon bug and consumed all the information he possibly could from books, magazines and online blogs. As a result of his reading and talking with fellow competitors he decided that he wanted to move to the next level and the best route to doing so was improving his strength and power.

When Andrew first came to the gym we went through a basic movement screen, and it quickly became clear that his body control through fundamental movements was poor and he also lacked flexibility. We agreed that Andrew's S&C was part of a long-term plan and therefore we would take an approach that built a solid foundation of athletic development and movement quality.

Andrew first came to see me in March, which was obviously coming into the triathlon season. Thankfully the type of work we were doing was not especially physically demanding as the focus was on technique and some injury prevention conditioning. As a result we were able to train through the season without fear of impairing performance. We decided that starting in March allowed us a good period of time to make the first season of S&C directed towards foundations for the following year. By the time winter training would come around in October we would have an excellent base to build on.

When we first met we went through a simple needs analysis process to determine how training would be directed. This was a combination of Andrew's own feelings about how he could improve and my observations of his qualities in the gym. As is generally the case, the two approaches matched up well. Although the swim was his weakest discipline this was generally down to lack of practice and technique, and so no particular discipline was targeted as a priority. His injury history was best described as having 'a few niggles'. He had not lost more than a few days at a time to injury, although the problems that he had could be traced back to movement issues seen in the gym. Thankfully a number of these would be addressed through our foundation of movement approach. The programme consisted of three main elements: movement control and preparation; whole body strength and patterning; and isolated conditioning.

Table 8.2 **Sample exercise regime for an absolute beginner**

Name: Andrew		Session Date: 22 March 2010		
Exercise	Comments	Sets	Reps	Weight
1a. Lunge walk		3	25 metres	30kg
1b. Spiderman crawl		3	15 metres	n/a
1c. Yoga sun salutation		3	n/a	n/a
2a. Step-ups		4	8	30kg
2b. Hop-stick		4	5	n/a
3a. Front squat		3	8	40kg
3b. Shoulder swimmers		3	15	n/a
4a. Side plank		3	40s	n/a
4b. Glute bridge		3	12	n/a
4c. Calf raise		3	12	n/a

CASE STUDY THE SECOND-SEASON TRAINER

Debbie was a pretty advanced trainer with a good background of gym work. She had been a good middle-distance runner in her youth during which time she had done a lot of athletics drills. Over the past 18 months she had also been carrying out a good progressive S&C regime, which had seen gains in both the gym and in her race times. She was highly motivated, but did not have a great deal of time to dedicate to her sessions.

The sample workout below is taken from January/February. Having built a good base of conditioning through the winter, the focus was on strength and power in the gym (these qualities will later be developed in more specific ways). There are relatively few exercises in the session, because the emphasis is on working very intensely on a few key movements. The session uses a 'complex training' type system, which pairs strength exercises with mechanically similar power exercises.

Table 8.3 **Sample exercise regime for a second-season trainer**

Name: Debbie		Session Date: 4 Jan 2009		
Exercise	Comments	Sets	Reps	Weight
Barbell mobility warm-up	Front squat, dead lift, clock lunge	3	10	20kg
1a. Box squats		5	5	75kg
1b. Rebound jumps		5	5	Body weight
2a. Single-leg squat off a box	Hold a med ball for weight	4	8	10kg
2b. Hop on to a box		4	5	Body weight
3a. Assisted pull-ups		4	5	n/a
3b. Med ball slams		4	5	6kg
4a. Aleknas		3	10	10kg
4b. Weighted plank		3	45 secs	15kg

CASE STUDY THE ADVANCED TRAINER

Adam was an elite triathlete competing at a national level and had medalled in several Ironman competitions. He ran his own business and was able to dedicate around 25 hours per week to triathlon. His performance gains had plateaued and it was clear that just adding more volume was no longer going to be the answer. This gave us the luxury of having complete freedom to write the perfect programme to suit him with almost no lifestyle constraints.

The programme featured below is taken from a pre-competition phase during April. The programme is split over a number of micro-sessions rather than large gym sessions.

Table 8.4	Sample exercise regime for an advanced trainer

Session 1 – Swim strength		Session Date: April		
Exercise	Comments	Sets	Reps	Dist.
1. Swimming drills set by coach	Use this session as part of a normal swim session, preferably speed sets. Take three mins recovery between sets			
2. Normal swim warm-up				
3. Bungee resisted swimming		4	5	25m

CASE STUDY THE ADVANCED TRAINER cont.

Session 2 – Cycle-specific strength		Session Date: April		
Exercise	Comments	Sets	Reps	Weight
10 mins progressive cycling warm-up	Either use a good (safe) hill or on a stationary bike, both in a high gear/resistance Cycle easy for 3 minutes between power sprints			
Dynamic flexibility if indoors				
Power sprints (10-sec max sprint, 50-sec recovery)		3	10	n/a
Finish with either short fast session or cool down				

Session 3 – Running mechanics and plyometrics		Session Date: April		
Exercise	Comments	Sets	Reps	Weight
Hurdle drills warm-up (choose three drills)	Perform this micro-session prior to a running speed workout. This will serve as great preparation and give the best transfer of training	3	6	n/a
1a. Skipping		3	30 metres	n/a
1b. A-march		3	20 metres	n/a
1c. Strides		3	50 metres	n/a
2. 60m sprints @ 80 per cent max.		1	10	n/a

Session 4 – Gym strength and power		Session Date: April		
Exercise	Comments	Sets	Reps	Weight
1. Dynamic flexibility warm-up		1	n/a	n/a
2. Jump squats		4	5	30kg
3a. Deep single-leg squats off box		3	8	5kg
3b. Lunge jumps		3	4	Body weight
4a. Roll-outs		3	8	n/a
4b. Clap press-ups		3	8	Body weight
5a. Hanging leg raises		3	12	n/a
5b. Weighted plank		6	15s	10

Session 5 – Prehab session		Session Date: April		
Exercise	Comments	Sets	Reps	Weight
1a. Face pulls	All exercises performed as a circuit. Perform 2–3 times per week at home	2–3	30s	n/a
1b. YTML		2–3	40s	n/a
1c. Dead bugs		2–3	40s	n/a
1d. Weighted glute bridge		2–3	20s	n/a
1e. Side lying leg raise		2–3	20s	n/a

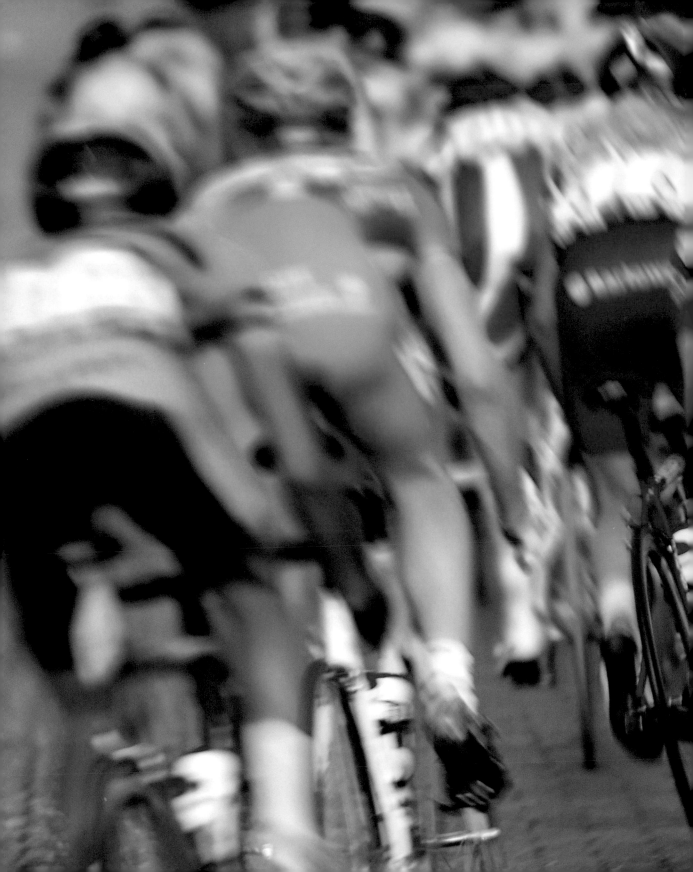

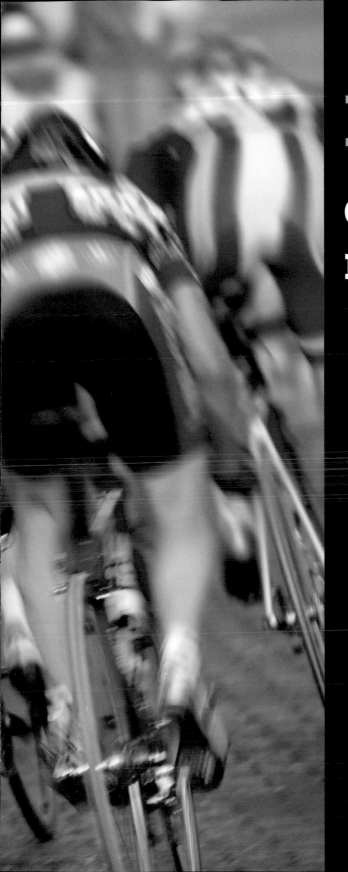

part 4
exercise
reference

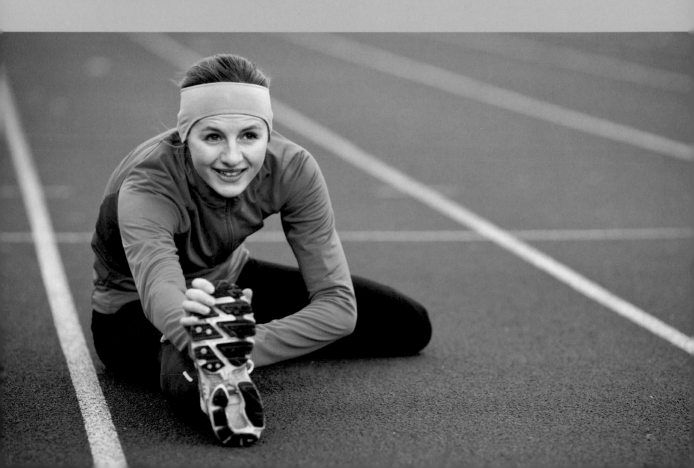

009
conditioning exercises

9.1 Introduction

This chapter serves as a reference for conditioning exercises. These are subdivided into leg and hip exercises, trunk work, movement control and shoulder work. Of course there are literally hundreds of exercises that can be used to achieve these goals and there is no way they can all be included in this book. However most of the fundamental 'families' of exercises are described,

so this collection will allow the athlete to compose a well-rounded conditioning regime.

Unlike strength exercises, which can be made harder or easier through the weight of the bar, conditioning exercises tend to have an inherent intensity. Therefore a very simplistic guide is given as to whether the movement is easy, medium or hard (or across a range if load can be added).

9.2 LEG AND HIP EXERCISES

Ex 9.1 Glute bridge

The glute bridge is an unavoidable classic, which addresses the hugely common problem of 'underactive glutes'. The main function of the glute (buttocks) is to extend the hip, which is exactly what this exercise does. It is important to make sure that you feel the work is coming from the glute and not the hamstring (back of thigh). In the case of the latter you will need to use a lower-intensity version of the movement until the glutes are performing correctly.

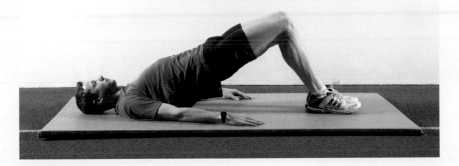

Key points
- Start with your hips on the floor and your knees bent to approx. 45 degrees
- Push your heels into the floor
- Consciously try to contract the glute
- Perform slowly and with control

Errors/Issues
- Hamstrings doing most of the work (This means the exercise level is too hard)

- Arching the lower back at the top of the movement

Progressions and variations
- Basic double-legged
- Double-legged with weight across the hips
- Single-legged
- Single-legged with weight across the hips

Ex 9.2 Fire hydrants

Unlike the glute bridge the fire hydrant exercise covers the other main function of the glute – external rotation – as well as hip extension. It also requires a good level of trunk control to keep the hips level and to avoid the back arching. Therefore while it is a fairly low-intensity exercise the fire hydrant is excellent for developing movement control around the trunk and pelvis.

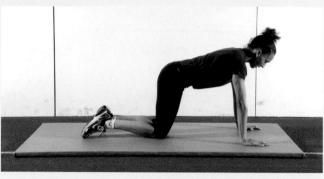

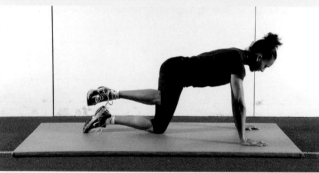

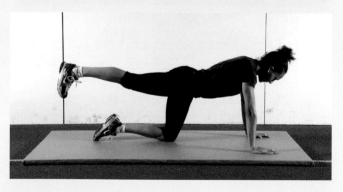

Key points
- Begin by opening the hip out sideways (see middle image)
- Next, extend the leg back fully, squeezing the glute as you do so
- Keep the hips level as you open the thigh
- Maintain a neutral spine as you extend the leg out

Errors/Issues
- Athletes often attempt to make up for weak or immobile hips through compensatory movements. This will lead only to the practice of poor movement and exacerbate the issue

Progressions and variations
- Small ankle weights may be used, but really this is best kept as a low-intensity control drill rather than making it high intensity

Ex 9.3 Band walks

This exercise targets the small glute medius, which lifts the leg out to the side of the body and is important for keeping the knee stable and avoiding 'dropping in'. Athletes tend to rate this highly because it induces a major burn in the glutes and so you definitely know it's working. The key is to make sure that the technique is tight, as small differences in posture can mean that very different muscles get worked.

Key points

- Keep feet wide apart and move sideways by pushing the knee outwards
- Adjust the difficulty through different thicknesses of band and adjusting the position on the leg (lower makes it harder)
- Stay tall

Errors/Issues

- Sitting back will cause the pelvis to change position and take the emphasis away from the glute medius
- Keep the torso upright – athletes often lean to the side to cheat the movement

Progressions and variations

- Manipulate distances walked and band position to avoid getting stale

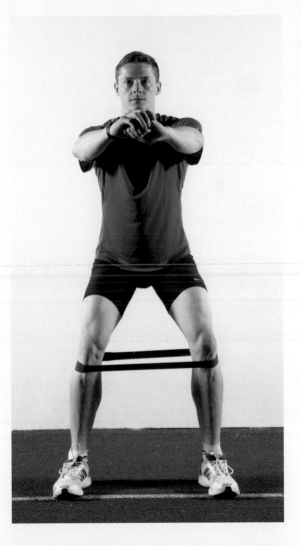

Ex 9.4 Calf raise (Gastrocnemius version)

The calf complex, including the Achilles tendon, can take quite a lot of abuse in a triathlete. The high volumes of cycling place a great demand on the muscle, and the tendon is key for producing elastic energy in running. The calf raise can help to improve the quality of both these tissues. Placing a greater emphasis on the eccentric phase (the descent) is a good way of ensuring against tendon problems, which many triathletes suffer from.

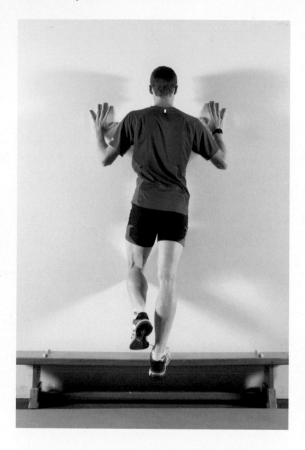 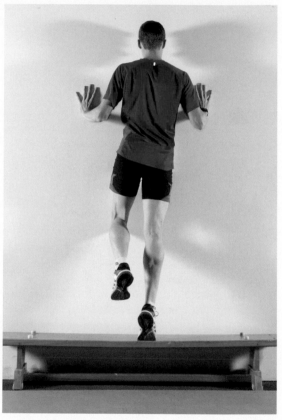

Key points
- Make sure only the ball of the foot is supported
- Work through a full range of motion up and down (unless this causes pain)

Errors/Issues
- Avoid rapid movements or holding on to supports excessively

Progressions and variations
- Single-leg version
- Eccentric – two feet up, one foot slowly down
- Add dumb-bells or kettlebells for extra load
- Use a leg press to add heavy load

Ex 9.5 Calf raise (Soleus version)

By performing the movement in a bent knee position the gastrocnemius is shortened, which means the emphasis is placed on the other major calf muscle – the soleus.

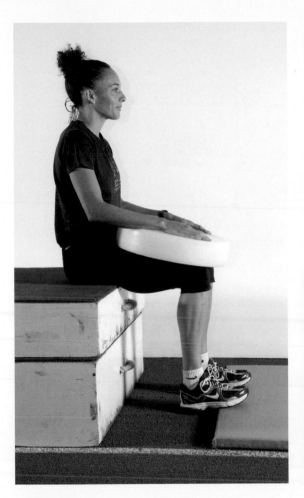
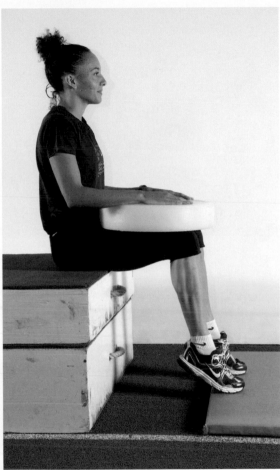

Key points
- Make sure only the ball of the foot is supported
- Work through a full range of motion, up and down (unless this causes pain)

Errors/Issues
- Avoid rapid movements or holding on to supports excessively

Progressions and variations
- To add load either place a weight on the knees or have a partner lean on you

Ex 9.6 Hamstring bridge

As a rule of thumb triathletes don't tend to suffer from hamstring injuries. However if you have sustained an injury in the past this may still come back to hamper your triathlon running. This simple exercise works effectively to strengthen the hamstrings through hip extension (which is what they do when running). However if you want stronger hamstrings for performance enhancement then the whole body barbell exercises in the strength and power section (*see* p. 154) are more suitable.

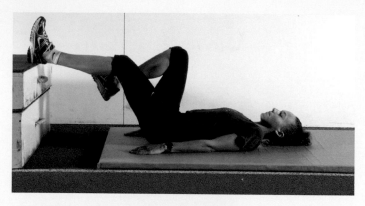

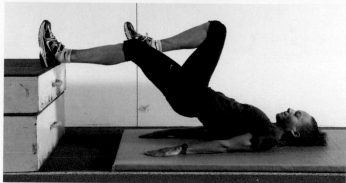

Key points
- Keep the movement slow and controlled and don't try to force out extra reps
  More TUT (time under tension) through the range is most important

Errors/Issues
- Make sure the opposite knee doesn't swing up to generate upward momentum to cheat
- Keep the active knee soft, not locked

Progressions and variations
- Double- or single-legged version
- Raise the height of the box or bench

Ex 9.7 Side lying leg raises

This is a very simple but effective exercise for targeting the glute medius. This is a muscle, which is often weak and has implications for control of the knee, particularly during running.

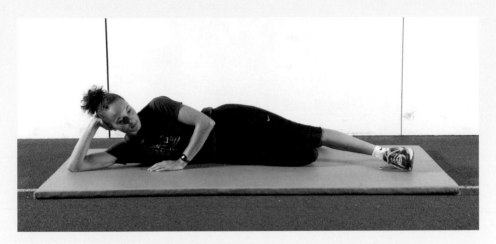

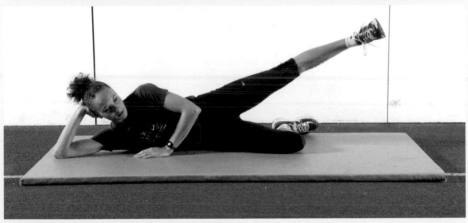

Key points
- Keep hips forward and lift from the side
- Perform slow controlled lifts

Errors/Issues
- Do not allow the hips to open out towards the ceiling

Progressions and variations
- Add light manual resistance or light ankle weights
- Add a hold and a small circular movement to increase work

Ex 9.8 Tibialis anterior raises

An important principle of training is that the body must be in balance. The tibialis anterior (the thin strip of muscle that runs down the front of the shin) may seem fairly insignificant. However if this is not kept in balance with calf development it can lead to big problems. This is a very simple exercise, which can be done between sets of bigger exercises, or even at home through the day.

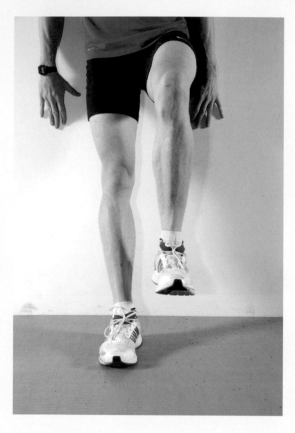 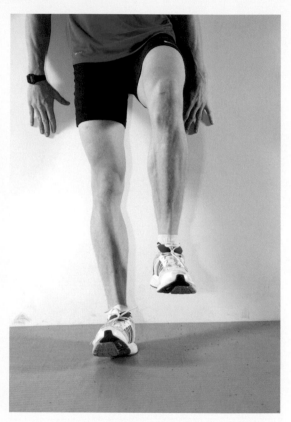

Key points
- Focus on time and quality rather than repetitions

Errors/Issues
- Make sure you control the eccentric – don't just let the toes drop without control

Progressions and variations
- Progress to a single-leg version

9.3 TRUNK CONDITIONING EXERCISES

Ex 9.9 Dead bugs

This is one of the most underrated exercises on the planet. It is ideal for developing the ability to move one arm and the opposite leg while keeping the trunk stable – in nutshell, exactly what we do when swimming, cycling and running!

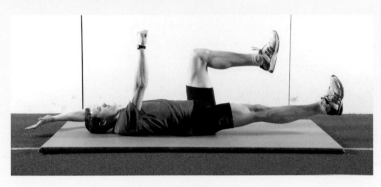

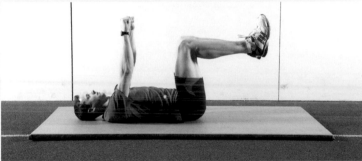

Key points
- One arm and the opposite leg are extended out, keeping close to the ground without touching
- The back must stay flat/neutral and not change shape from the start position
- Try to keep the pelvis 'tucked in' with the lower abdominals
- Movements must be slow and controlled

Errors/Issues
- The back position cannot be maintained
- The work feels as if it is coming from the back rather than the abdomen

Progressions and variations
- Hold a light weight in each hand (1–2.5kg)
- Hold the end position for 10–30 seconds
- Add ankle weights (1–2kg)

Ex 9.10 Aleknas

The alekna (named after a famous thrower credited with inventing this exercise) is essentially a more challenging version of the dead bug. Although it lacks the specific diagonal pattern that the dead bug offers, it makes up for it with the high-level challenge it places on the ability to hold a neutral spine.

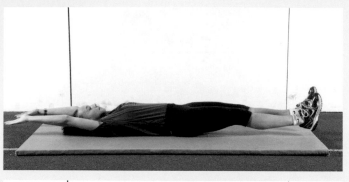

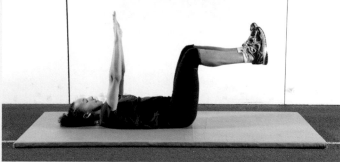

Key points
- Extend both arms and legs, keeping close to the ground without touching
- The back must stay flat/neutral and not change shape from the start position
- Try to keep the pelvis 'tucked in' with the lower abdominals
- Movements must be slow and controlled

Errors/Issues
- The back position cannot be maintained
- The work feels as if it is coming from the back rather than the abdomen

Progressions and variations
- If too difficult the exercise can be regressed by shortening the range of movement and gradually extended over time
- Hold a light weight in the hands
- Place a weight on the shins as well as in the hands (maximum 10kg each end)
- Hold the end position for 10–30 seconds (without weights)

Ex 9.11 The plank

In recent years this exercise has become extremely popular. It is an excellent tool for developing stability through the trunk, as it is based on preventing movement. However while it is frequently used it is also often abused. Make sure that the work is directed to the mid-section and that form is perfect. Too often athletes adopt horrendous positions in an attempt to rack up the longest plank they can – quality definitely beats quantity.

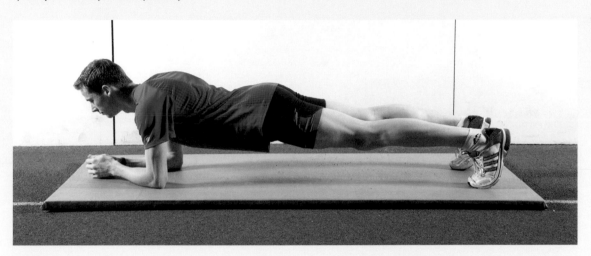

Key points

- Keep body parallel to the floor, with hips level
- Shoulders must be relaxed and not rounded
- Treat 60 seconds as the maximum time; if it is easy, move to a harder progression
- If the work feels like it is coming from the lower back then it is too hard

Errors/Issues

- Lifting hips
- Sagging hips
- Bracing shoulders to take the load

Progressions and variations

- Start with a basic plank for 30 seconds; if this is too hard, go from the knees
- 3-point plank: one arm or leg is removed from the floor while staying level
- 2-point plank: one arm and the opposite leg are removed from the floor
- Marching plank: feet are alternately lifted slowly 3–5cm from the floor
- Weighted plank: a light to moderate weight (5–20kg) is placed across the hips during a basic plank

Ex 9.12 Side plank

Although it shares a common name with the plank, the side plank should be considered separately as the focus is distinctly different. To have a truly stable trunk we need to be able to stabilise from all angles and this includes side flexion (think of the cyclist rocking from side to side). The exercise not only targets the trunk but also the hips, and it can help to improve knee stability.

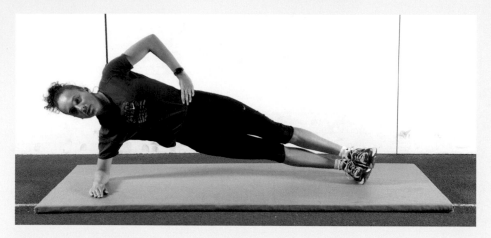

Key points
- Keep shoulders, hips and ankles all in line
- Exercise should stress the mid-section; if the shoulder is burning then move to an easier version

Errors/Issues
- Shoulder hitching up towards ear
- Hips either sagging or fixed higher than neutral

Progressions and variations
- Start with a side plank with knee on the floor and progress to feet on floor
- Add slow leg lifts (top leg raised towards ceiling then lowered)
- Partner resisted – partner applies small amount of downward pressure to the hips

Ex 9.13 Roll-outs

This is a tough exercise but an equally effective one. Similar to aleknas it requires the ability to keep the trunk fixed while the arms are moving. It also works the serratus anterior very effectively, which is an important muscle for controlling the position of the scapula. Therefore this is a fantastic exercise for improving swimming trunk strength.

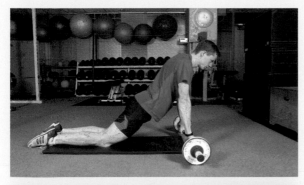

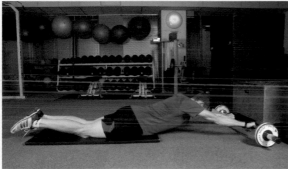

Key points
- Slowly roll the barbell forwards allowing your hands to move out in front of the body
- Work at a level that allows you to perform the movement to its full range
- Keep the elbows slightly soft
- There should be a straight line from the shoulder to the knee throughout (don't let the hips flex)

Errors/Issues
- Stop or regress the exercise if the back hurts or it feels as if this is where the work is coming from

Progressions and variations
- Begin with a barbell and perform the exercise from the knees
- A slightly easier but more functional version can be performed with dumb-bells, rolling each arm out alternately
- For a highly advanced version perform either of the above from the feet

Ex 9.14 Superman

While the previous exercises are excellent for developing the capacity of the trunk, the Superman is all about control. The movement itself is not taxing but control of posture requires a great deal of concentration. Therefore it is useful if possible to use a mirror or have someone watch you. Don't be afraid to be ruthlessly perfectionist with this one – quality is everything!

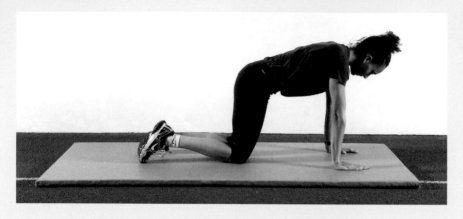

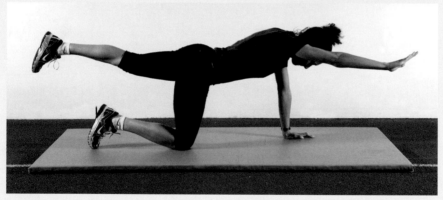

Key points
- Move slowly with control
- Make sure you get some form of feedback as to how you are moving
- Extend one arm and the opposite leg while keeping the trunk stable throughout

Errors/Issues
- The back should not arch at all from its original position
- There should be no twisting through the spine/trunk

Progressions and variations
- None – just aim to perform this movement perfectly with total consistency

Ex 9.15 Prone extension hold

Specific lower-back training is often uncalled for as sufficient work can be achieved during whole body exercises such as squats. However if this is a particular area of weakness or the athlete is not doing whole body strength movements then this can help to give a more rounded trunk training regime.

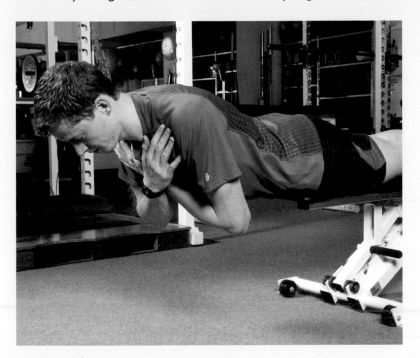

Key points

- Have a partner sit on your legs to secure you
- Line up so that the top of the hips just come off the bench
- Keep torso level with the floor, looking downwards
- Keep to a maximum of 90 seconds

Errors/Issues

- Beware of excessively arching the back
- Once position drops, terminate the exercise
- Stop immediately if pain is experienced

Progressions and variations

- Extend arms in front
- Hold a weights disc (2.5–10kg) across your chest

Ex 9.16 Woodchop

Rotational exercises are often ignored or at best under-represented in most training programmes. However given that all three triathlon disciplines involve alternate use of the limbs and therefore the control of rotational forces, they should be considered a fundamental. Although the woodchop is a dynamic movement it is performed slowly, so the focus is more on controlling the rotation than producing it powerfully.

Key points
- Hips should remain facing forwards at all times with the movement coming from the chest and shoulders (thorax)
- Move in a controlled manner from the hip diagonally across the opposite shoulder

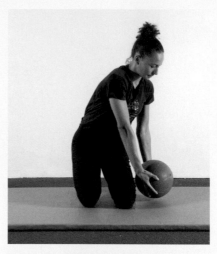

Errors/Issues
- Avoid arching the back at the top of the movement or rounding at the bottom to gain a greater range of movement
- Arms should remain pointing in the same direction as the chest and not come across the body
- Keep the movement controlled at all times and do not try to force the end of range

Progressions and variations
- Stick to moderate loads up to a maximum of 10kg (either med ball or disc). Alternatively cable pulley machines can be used effectively, particularly hydraulic resistance machines
- Can be performed from standing or on knees

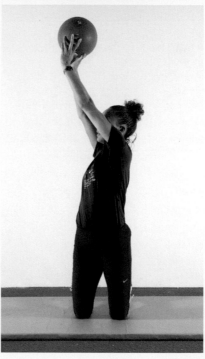

Ex 9.17 Rolling

This may get some strange looks at the health club, but it is a superb exercise for improving trunk control in swimming. It also serves as a good test of trunk control. Rolling is not a high-intensity exercise, but requires high levels of skill and control.

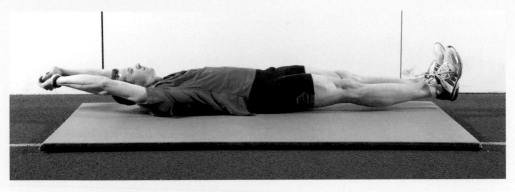

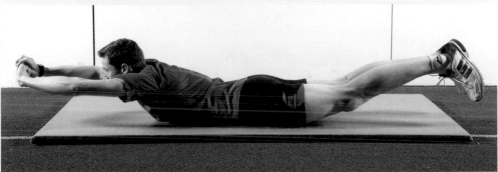

Key points
- Start by lying on your back and slowly roll to one side, then on to your front
- The movement should involve all body parts rolling simultaneously with full control at all times

Errors/Issues
- Look out for one body part (e.g. shoulders) 'leading' the movement
- There should be no jerky movements and you should not drop at any point

Progressions and variations
- Aim to perfect your control. Once you have done so you can revisit this exercise intermittently to ensure that you have kept in touch with this skill

Ex 9.18 Swiss ball Russian twist

Although this can be looked on as something of a relic from the obsession with Swiss balls and core stability in the late 1990s it actually offers several useful benefits. As well as working the obliques through the rotational movement it also requires the athlete to keep the hips and lower back stable. This helps to promote the ability to dissociate between the hip, lower and upper back, which we have learned is important in swimming skills. Furthermore we get a free workout for the glutes and hamstrings, which are working to keep the hips elevated.

Key points

- Hips up and parallel to the floor
- Shoulders, neck and head are supported by the ball
- The ball should roll from between the shoulder blades to the outside of the upper arm

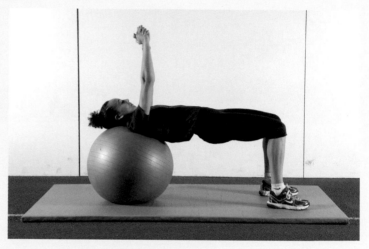

Errors/Issues

- It is possible to cheat this by moving the arms to the side without rolling the shoulder
- Try to keep the rotation in the upper back and shoulders, and not in the lower back

Progressions and variations

- Start with no weight and slowly introduce light loads (5–10kg dumb-bell)
- If you are very advanced you may be able to lift the leg (on the side you are turning) off the floor

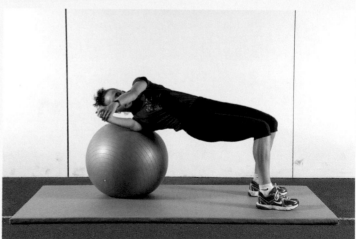

Ex 9.19 Double leg lowers

This is a challenging exercise that is often used as a test of an athlete's capacity to hold the trunk stable while moving the legs.

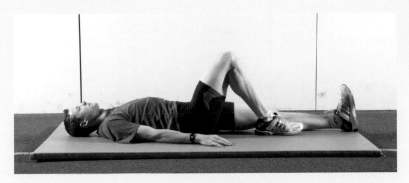

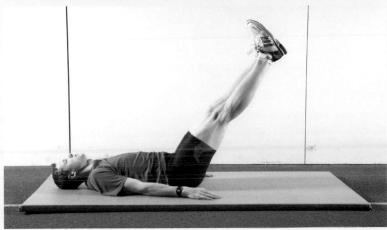

Key points

- Line up by placing one ankle level with the opposite knee then bring both feet level, extending the legs to give you the start position
- Stop the exercise if you feel pain and/or cannot keep your lower back flat to the floor
- The legs are then slowly lowered to just above the floor, being kept straight throughout before returning to the start

Errors/Issues

- Avoid bouncing feet off the floor
- Form must be kept intact throughout

Progressions and variations

- Can be progressed to variations of hanging leg raises (*see* below)

Ex 9.20 Hanging leg raises

These can be performed using anything you can hang from, including wall bars or a chin-up bar. The exercise can also be made slightly easier using a Roman chair. This challenging exercise is excellent for athletic development.

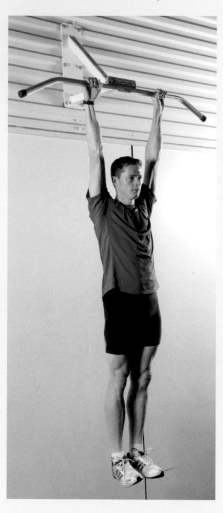

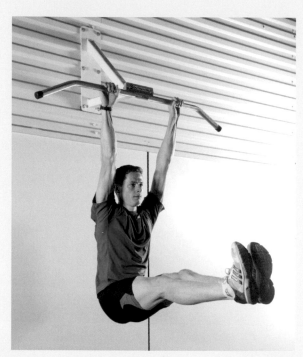

Key points
- The pelvis should roll backwards with the movement
- Keep slow and controlled for effective development, particularly during the descent

Errors/Issues
- Beware of using the arms to 'cheat' the movement
- If it feels as if the work is coming from the hip flexors regress the intensity and focus on rolling the pelvis

Progressions and variations
- Begin with a bent knee version
- Progress to straight legs, with the ultimate aim being to get feet to hands
- All versions can also be intensified by hold a med ball between the feet or knees, which also works the adductors

9.4 MOVEMENT QUALITY DEVELOPMENT

Ex 9.21 Lunge walk

This is one of the most commonly used warm-up exercises. It is no wonder, because a whole host of important elements can be developed. As a result there are many variations on the standard exercise. Lunge walking helps to mobilise the hips, develop knee stability and by retaining posture we are able to develop trunk control. Be wary though – the range of movement and eccentric stress of landing can cause the uninitiated to become very sore. Start off with small amounts and gradually progress over the weeks.

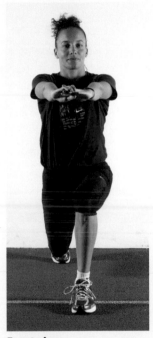

Front view

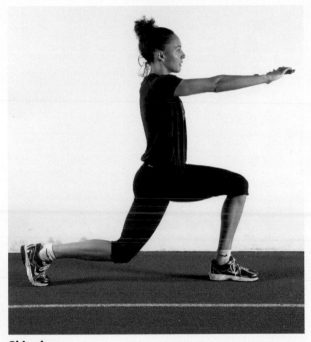

Side view

Key points
- Focus on control at all times
- Keep the whole of the front foot on the floor when pulling through for the next step

Errors/Issues
- Knees 'falling in'
- Loss of control in the upper body – should remain tall and strong and avoid leaning back, falling to the side, etc

Progressions and variations
- Reverse lunge
- Clock lunge
- Lunge with side flexions

Ex 9.22 Hop-stick (also known as Hop and hold)

The hop-stick is a classic exercise for developing what S&C coaches call 'load acceptance'. While single-leg strength exercises develop the strength to hold the knee in position when running, hop-stick work will develop the coordination and control to fire the muscles during the brief period that the foot is in contact with the ground. Control and quality are everything with this work. Try to use a wide number of variations in order to make sure that the learning stimulus is kept fresh.

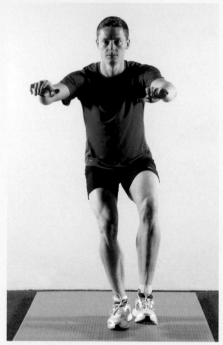

View from the front

Key points
- Work to a level that is challenging but can be controlled: if too easy the exercise will not provide a challenge; if too tough it will not give you a chance to control the movement
- Maintain excellent posture and stay relaxed; avoid rounding the back and becoming overly tense
- Flat foot landing

Errors/Issues
- Knees 'falling in'
- Landing on toes/front of foot
- Excessive tension through upper body
- Failure to 'stick the landing' – i.e., double-bounce

Progressions and variations
- Start with a basic left–right–left
- Gradually increase the distance of the hop
- Also use same leg to same leg variation
- Introduce diagonal and rotational hops to mix things up

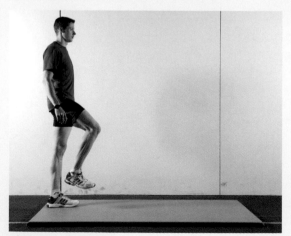

View from the side A

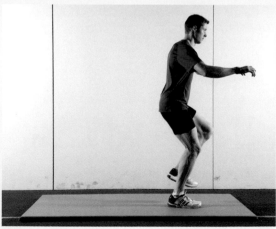

View from the side B

Ex 9.23 Spiderman crawl

This somewhat novel exercise is a hugely effective and efficient warm-up activity that gives lots of bang for your buck. In addition to the primary benefit of improving mobility around the hips prior to training, the crawl also helps to improve shoulder and trunk stability. There is even a theory among developmental psychologists that performing primal infantile movements such as this can 'prime the brain' to be in a state of readiness to learn. On this basis they offer added benefit before special strength sessions or skill drills that involve motor learning.

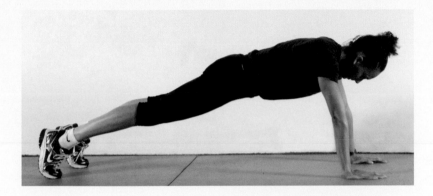

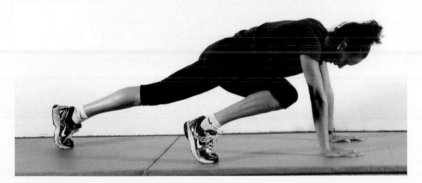

Key points

- Look to work through a full range of motions in each exercise without straining excessively or losing form
- Concentrate on keeping the shoulders set and the spine in neutral

Errors/Issues

- Try to avoid rounding the back and make sure the knee goes outside the elbow

Progressions and variations

- Start off working over 5–10m and gradually build up to around 20m
- Combine crawl series for a greater conditioning stress

Ex 9.24 Downward dog

Yoga is a fantastic way of stretching the hamstrings and calves (the back chain). When stretching these areas the aim is to stress the muscles at the back of the legs while keeping the lower back flat/neutral. However far too often the lower back becomes rounded in an attempt to 'cheat' more movement. The downward dog provides a great way to stretch the nerves (often overlooked) and even adds an element of shoulder stability work.

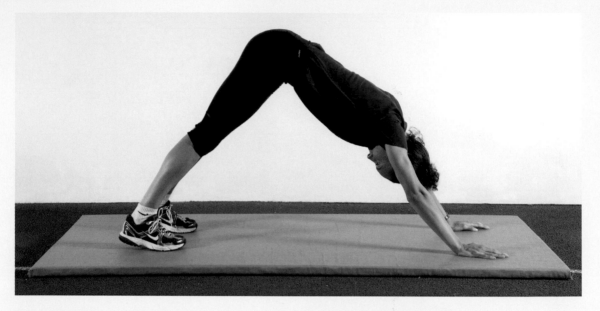

Key points

- Perform the exercise at a level you can manage with good technique; use blocks to raise your hands if need be
- Continually monitor your form: heels down, knees pushed back, back flat and neck relaxed

Errors/Issues

- Don't bounce or force the positions

Progressions and variations

- Progress the duration you hold the pose
- Start to incorporate into routines to add a conditioning component

Ex 9.25 Sun salutation

One of the issues that prevents many triathletes from regularly utilising the benefits of yoga is the time factor. With three disciplines, plus strength and conditioning, the idea of adding a 90-minute yoga class is completely impractical. A great way of getting a bite-sized element of yoga into your training is the sun salutation, which involves a rounded series of mobility challenges combined with a good level of muscle conditioning. The series itself can be quite complex and the coaching of its intricacies is beyond this book. Therefore you should seek a yoga teacher to learn a sequence that is appropriate for your level.

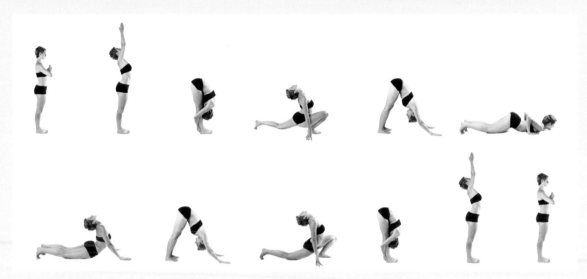

Key points

- Only perform movements you can execute properly – incorrect shapes are ineffective and dangerous
- Perform regularly before gym sessions to make steady progress and also gain an excellent warm-up

Errors/Issues

- The most important point is to only attempt elements of the pose which you can do comfortably and correctly

Progressions and variations

- There are many variations on this theme, try to find one which is best suited to your ability

Ex 9.26 Thoracic extension mobiliser

One of the most common side effects of modern life is thoracic stiffness (lack of mobility in the vertebrae of the upper back), as discussed in chapter 3. This can have direct performance implications such as the inability to execute the swim stroke efficiently. It may also have implications for injury risk as the lack of movement must be compensated for by other areas such as the lower back and the shoulder. This exercise can be performed either with a foam roller or two tennis balls in a sports sock. Each of these works slightly differently: the foam roller helps to open the joints, whereas the tennis balls release tension in the surrounding tissue. Therefore using both methods give better overall results.

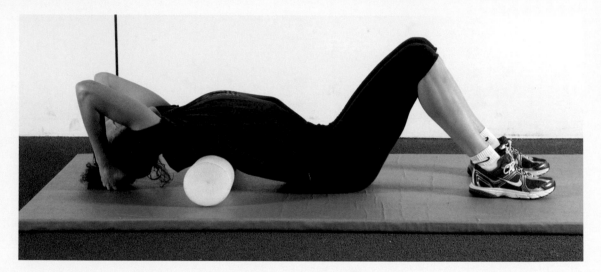

Key points
- Position the foam roller/tennis balls between two vertebrae around the bottom of the rib cage
- Deliberately arch the spine over the implement, aiming to open the specific area being worked
- Repeat 1–2 times and then move up to the next vertebrae

Errors/Issues
- *Always* keep this technique to the upper back only; avoid the lower back and the neck

Progressions and variations
- n/a

Ex 9.27 Indian sitting

While the foam roller and tennis ball work help to improve thoracic extension, Indian sitting exercises target rotation and lateral flexion.

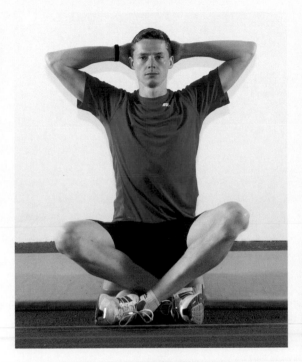 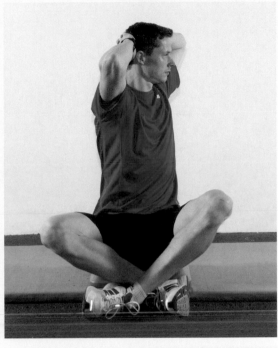

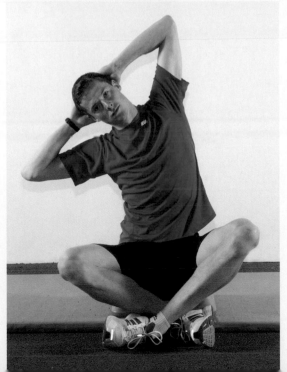

Key points
- Sit on a cushion or block that enables you to sit cross-legged with a flat back (if the back is rounded then raise the block)
- Perform rotations and side flexions separately

Errors/Issues
- Avoid rounding the back or excessively forcing the range of movement

Progressions and variations
- n/a

Ex 9.28 Scorpions

This is another exercise that helps to mobilise the spine and improve overall mobility. These types of movement are particularly important for 'resetting the body' after long periods of sitting, such as desk work or driving.

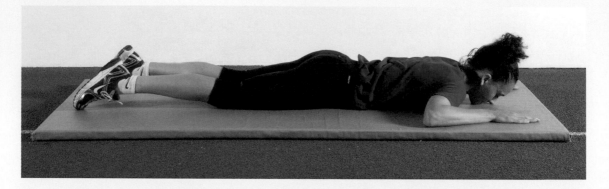

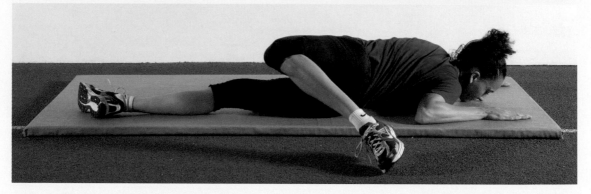

Key points
- Keep the shoulders on the floor and allow the hips to roll
- Gradually build the range of movement through the sets

Errors/Issues
- Don't try to force the movement
- Make sure rolling comes through the upper rather than lower back

Progressions and variations
- n/a

Ex 9.29 Foam roller ITB

One of the most common issues and movement dysfunctions that triathletes exhibit is ITB (iliotibial band) syndrome, which can lead to this long tendon pulling the kneecap out of line (patella tracking). Continuing to train through this problem can be very painful and lead to serious damage to the knee. Releasing tension in the ITB with a foam roller is a painful but very effective method of alleviating this issue.

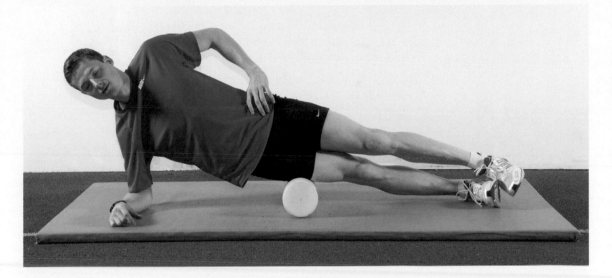

Key points
- Place the foam roller on the outside of the thigh and allow a little body weight to be applied into the roller
- Start close to the thigh and gradually move downwards
- Find the areas that are most sensitive and concentrate on them

Errors/Issues
- n/a

Progressions and variations
- Ultimately this is a short-term fix and needs to be combined with an exercise programme that strengthens the hips and restores muscle balance

Ex 9.30 Towel scrunches

We have already learned that the feet are ignored at an athlete's peril. This is a simple exercise that works the intrinsic muscles of the foot, which keep it healthy and promote the natural elastic mechanics of its design.

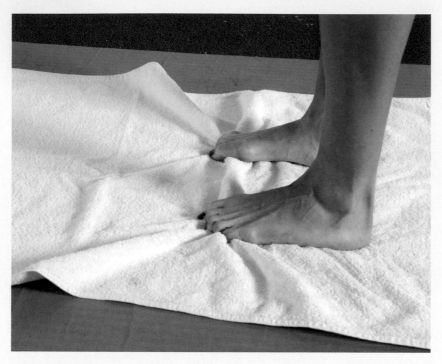

Key points
- Curl the toes to drag the towel towards you
- Work slowly through a full range, including when straightening the toes

Errors/Issues
- Focus on working for increasing time periods (30–90 seconds) rather than reps

Progressions and variations
- This is just the tip of the iceberg for footwork. Barefoot exercises in sand (pit, or beach if you're lucky) are another great option

Ex 9.31 Hip flexor stretch

The hip flexors at the front of the hip can easily become shortened and tight due to the amount of sitting we do. This simple stretch is excellent for opening out the hips before a session.

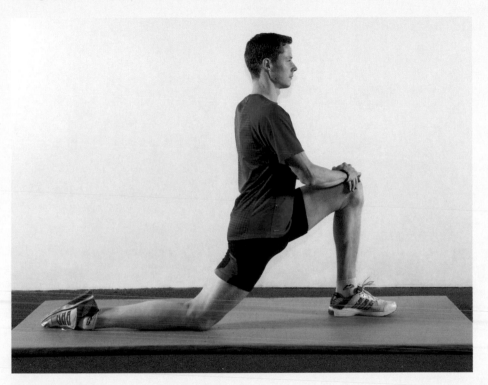

Key points

- Use the initial lunge position to open out the front of the hip. This will hit the iliacus portion of the hips
- Add the side lean towards the lead leg to stretch the psoas

Errors/Issues

- Make sure posture remains tall and allow the hips to sink towards the floor

Progressions and variations

- This can be done statically or adapted into a lunge walk to provide a more dynamic warm-up activity

Ex 9.32 Hamstring march

The hamstrings are probably the most commonly stretched muscle group. Static stretching of the hamstrings is of questionable benefit, and many common stretches are performed poorly and actually just open out the lower back. The hamstring march is excellent for opening the muscles and nerves of the hamstrings and, if performed correctly, will help to improve control of the hips and back.

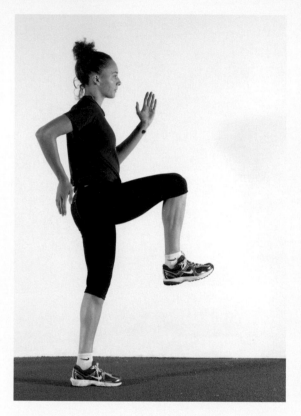 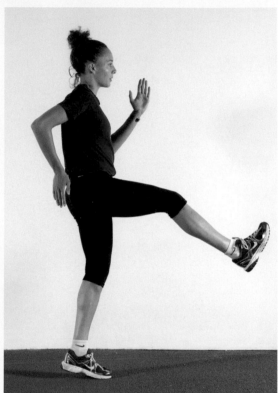

Key points
- Start by lifting the thigh, then extend the knee
- Keep the toes pulled up towards the shin

Errors/Issues
- The back *must* be kept in neutral. Avoid rounding the back in order to try cheating some apparent extra range in the march

Progressions and variations
- This can start as a controlled walk and gradually be advanced into a skip

Ex 9.33 Walking glute stretch

This is another good dynamic movement to do when the hips can become tight. It opens up the hips while helping to warm up at the same time.

Key points

- Staying tall, hug the knee into the chest as you slowly walk
- Alternate legs with each step

Errors/Issues

- Pull the thigh towards you, rather than the other way around

Progressions and variations

- n/a

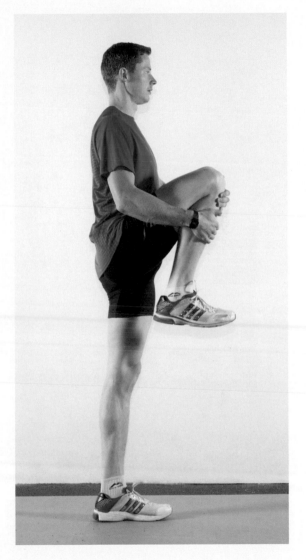

Ex 9.34 Ankle rolls

This is a very simple exercise, which can be used to achieve multiple goals. In addition to mobilising the ankle it should improve balance and control around the hips, knees and ankles as well as the muscles in the feet. All of these benefits will be increased further if the exercise is performed in bare feet.

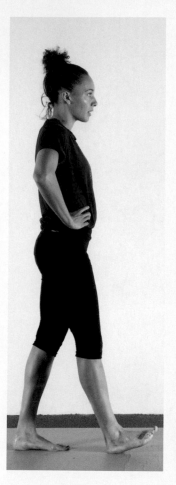 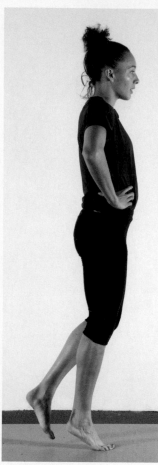

Key points
* Slowly roll with full control from the heel through to the big toe

Errors/Issues
* Look for and avoid any points where control is lost and the foot 'collapses'
* Keep the rest of the body tall and loose; avoid becoming rigid in search of balance

Progressions and variations
* n/a

9.5 SHOULDER PREHAB

Ex 9.35 YTML

YTML are the shapes made by the arms during the four movements. This is actually several exercises in one but when combined they take the shoulder through pretty much all of its fundamental movement patterns. Therefore the old cliché that if you do only one exercise for shoulder health make it this one, is probably true. The emphasis is on programming good movement patterns and fine control around the shoulder. Therefore this is also a good pre-swim warm-up exercise as it may improve fine motor control during the session

Key points
- Each part of the movement begins and ends with the start position
- Technique is everything with these movements – the idea is to train the correct movement pattern and so focus is vital
- If in doubt, do fewer reps if fatigue starts to cause a loss of form
- All movements should be performed slowly and deliberately

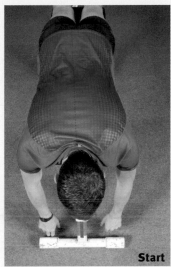
Start

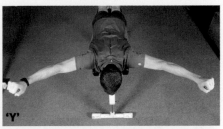
'Y'

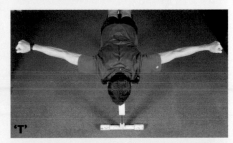
'T'

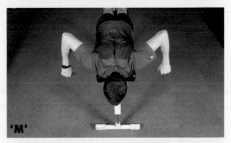
'M'

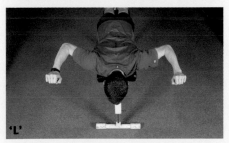
'L'

Errors/Issues
- Allowing the shoulders to 'hitch' up towards the ears
- Throwing the arms into each action to make it easier
- Cheating to get extra range of movement by using compensatory patterns

Progressions and variations
- Very light weights (1.25kg) can be used to enhance the exercise
- Change the order of performance, sometimes perform all of the Y's, all of the T's, etc. Other times perform one of each in sequence

Ex 9.36 Swimmers

Named for obvious reasons, this exercise is great for firing up the scapular retractors, which pull our shoulders back. It is rare to find an individual who does not need this type of work. You may find this is particularly useful after a long session in the saddle, when the back has been rounded and the shoulders pushed forwards. As well as improving shoulder health, this exercise is also important for helping to open out the chest to allow the powerful swimming muscles to work to their optimum level of function.

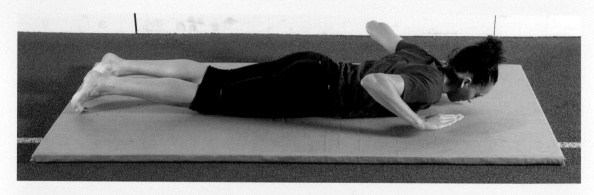

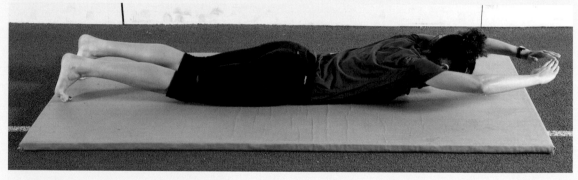

Key points
- Actively squeeze the shoulder blades back and lift hands off the floor
- Reach out to stretch the arms and gain a full range of movement

Errors/Issues
- Lifting the chest off the floor to assist
- Lifting head to look forwards (keep looking down)

Progressions and variations
- Add light weights (1.25–2.5kg)
- TUT (time under tension) is more important than reps here so work slowly for a set period of time rather than rushing to finish reps

Ex 9.37 Scap press-ups

The scap press-up is a fantastic exercise for working a muscle called the serratus anterior. This is important for keeping the shoulder blade flat to the rib cage and avoiding so-called 'winging', which can increase the risk of shoulder impingement. As well as working this muscle, the exercise is also good for teaching the ability to control the movements of the shoulder rather than using gross movements of the upper back.

Key points
- From press-up position allow the chest to drop and the shoulder blades to pinch together, then round the upper back to push them far apart
- This movement should come only from the upper back and nowhere else

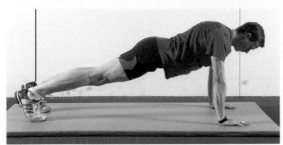

View from the side

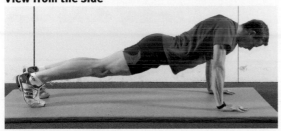

Errors/Issues
- It can feel strange performing such a small movement, so athletes are often tempted to compensate by flexing and extending their upper back

Progressions and variations
- If you struggle to control the movement or fatigue through holding the position then regress to a press-up from knees position
- Some athletes with a history of shoulder injury may still struggle and need to lean against a wall in a standing position
- For those who find it easy a weight can be placed across the shoulders (5–20kg) or a partner can apply resistance

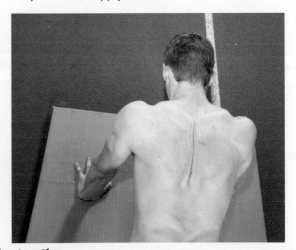

View from the top – notice the shoulder blades pinching together

Ex 9.38 Single-leg PNF pulls

This is actually a slightly novel version of a basic proprioceptive neuromuscular facilitation (PNF) pull. By performing it on one leg training is more efficient, because the glutes also get a workout and anti-rotational trunk control is also developed. However if your main focus is the shoulder and this version is too challenging, then go back to both feet on the ground. The PNF movement itself is a diagonal pattern across the body, which incorporates all of the major shoulder muscles. Ideally you can use elastic bands or hydraulic resistance machines, but a traditional cable stack machine or even a light disc will also work.

Key points
- The hand should move from the opposite hip in a diagonal path across the body
- The hand should take the furthest possible path across the body
- Keep the arm straight at all times

Errors/Issues
- Make sure as closely as possible the hand finishes at 45°

Progressions and variations
- Regress to double foot if necessary
- To challenge balance more, move to standing on the foot of the side you are pulling from

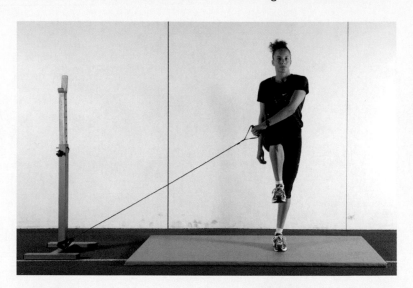

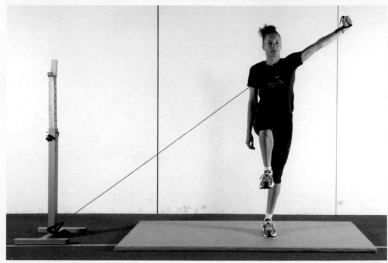

Ex 9.39 Face pulls

This is another shoulder exercise that requires elastic tubing but can also be performed using a cable stack. Face pulls are good for developing the strength of the shoulder retractors. The essence of it is pretty simple as the clue is in the title!

Key points
- Keep hands close together and pull in a controlled manner

Errors/Issues
- Keep shoulders 'set' and avoid hitching up towards ears

Progressions and variations
- The exercise itself remains pretty constant but can vary in load considerably. Light loads with elastic are good for training the movement, whereas heavier loads with weights will help to develop strength

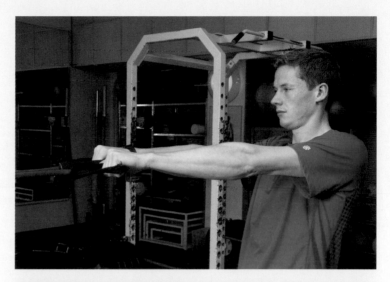

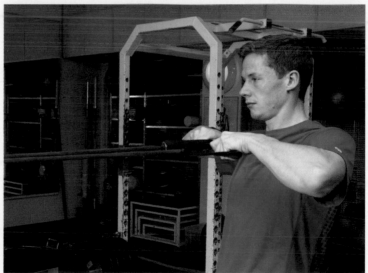

Ex 9.40 Bruce Lees

I must confess to being guilty of giving this exercise its slightly dubious name! Regardless of the title though it is an effective movement for developing both strength and control of the shoulder. The key is to keep the movements within the exercise distinct: first pull the shoulder back; then pull the elbow back; and finish with a rotation. This is certainly a more thorough approach than the 'physio's favourite', the external rotation, which is a very one-dimensional exercise.

Key points

- Start with the shoulder pulled forwards. Begin by pulling the shoulder back; next pull the elbow back as far as possible. Finally, rotate the forearm to a vertical position without letting the upper arm drop
- Keep as three separate movements

Errors/Issues

- Don't let the elbow drop during the rotation
- Make sure the shoulder stays set

Progressions and variations

- For strength gains, an elastic resistance band should be used; however this is also a good control exercise if performed unresisted and can be included as part of a pre-swim warm-up

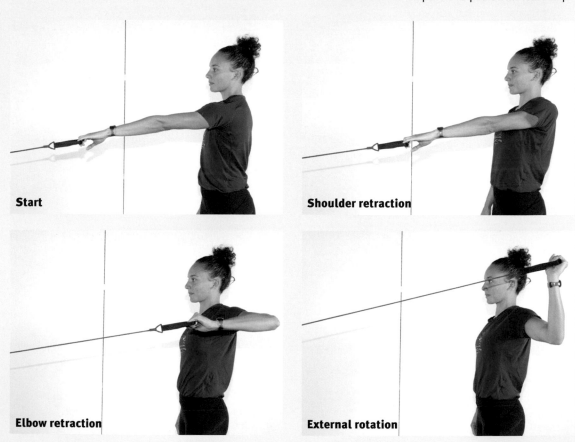

Start

Shoulder retraction

Elbow retraction

External rotation

Ex 9.41 Stick dislocations

These have a slightly different emphasis to the previous exercises in that the focus is on improving shoulder mobility rather than strength or control. As such it is probably most suitable for pre-swim sessions, pre-gym sessions or post-bike sessions.

Key points

- Start with a very wide grip and ease your way into the movement

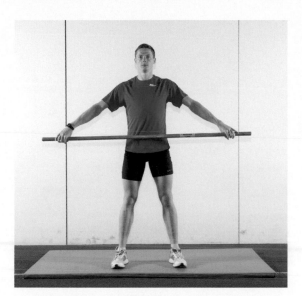

Errors/Issues

- Make sure the arms stay straight
- Don't force it! This should be comfortable and should never be painful or hard work

Progressions and variations

- Dislocations can be performed with a stick, a rope or a rubber band
- Progression is based on mobility and is measured by how close the hands are held together

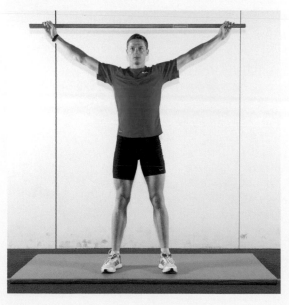

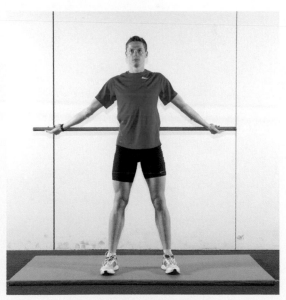

010
strength and power exercises

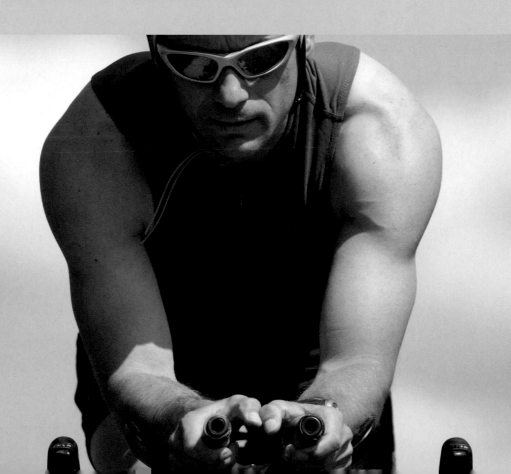

10.1 Introduction

This chapter deals with exercises that are naturally suitable for developing strength and power. The true value of these exercises lies in the fact that they are based on fundamental movement patterns such as squatting, lunging, pressing and pulling. This means that developing excellent control, then adding strength and power, is most likely to transfer to athletic performance in these types of activity. The exercises have the capacity to be heavily loaded. This means that they can induce a very significant training stimulus, which can have a profound effect on movement quality and capacity. However be wary of the temptation to load too quickly. Developing absolute excellence in movement will be the most fruitful path to increased athleticism, but only the smartest coaches and athletes are able to stick faithfully to this philosophy. In my experience 90 per cent of athletes load the movements too heavily, too quickly.

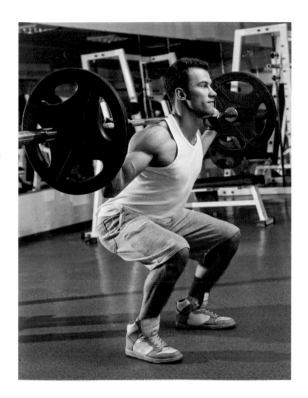

The power exercises offer more dynamic explosive options than the traditional movement patterns. Do not rush into these, because without strength there can be no power.

10.2 General strength
Bilateral squat patterns

The squat is one of the key fundamental movement patterns and is often used by S&C coaches as the starting point for an assessment of an athlete's movement ability. The movement has several derivatives including the front squat and the back squat (describing the position of the bar in relation to the body). It is also somewhat unusual in that, unlike most exercises, it is often performed through only a partial range of motion. There are a number of factors that influence the choice of squat and the depth of movement. (*see* chapter 5).

However I would urge athletes to focus on developing a good range of squat and strong technique before concentrating on strength development. By developing a good deep squat you will be able to unlock the potential for power in your hips and will produce stronger more stable knees (contrary to mythology, which warns against deep squatting).

Treating squats as a 'leg exercise' does them a great injustice. They are a whole body movement and develop mobility, trunk strength and body awareness. Therefore they are a staple in training. Occasionally an athlete may have an issue that makes squatting contra-indicated, such as disc herniation. For these athletes the leg press may be used as an alternative. It may also help the athlete who needs greater leg strength but whose squatting is limited by trunk strength.

The squat is a hugely versatile exercise that can be manipulated in many ways. This is vital as some form of squatting is ever-present in programming and so variety is essential:

- Light, full range squats can be used to develop mobility and athletic balance.

- The addition of a pause at the bottom of the movement, such as in a box squat, makes the movement much harder. Here a powerful drive is required to overcome the initial inertia and so the squat becomes more explosive. Similarly the addition of chains or rubber bands to the bar alter the weight of the bar, so that it becomes heavier towards the top of the movement.

- Jump squatting with a light to moderate bar is another way of developing explosive power.

Key squatting technique points
Each of the squat variations has its own specific technical points. However there are a number of elements that are consistent throughout all squatting patterns:

- The movement should be initiated by sitting the hips backwards. The knees will bend automatically, but starting with the hips will ensure a balance between these two key joints.

- Keep the back tight with the abs braced and do not allow the back to round at all. If the lower back starts to round you have gone too low, the weight is too heavy or basic technique and control need work.

- The knees must remain stable and in line with the toes (i.e., not 'falling in').

- Tempo will vary according to the goals of the session (*see* below), but the descent should always be controlled and the athlete should never 'bounce' out of the bottom.

- Feet should be around shoulder width apart but most importantly you should feel comfortable.

- Weight should be evenly distributed across the whole foot, not allowing it to shift to the front of the foot or roll inwardly.

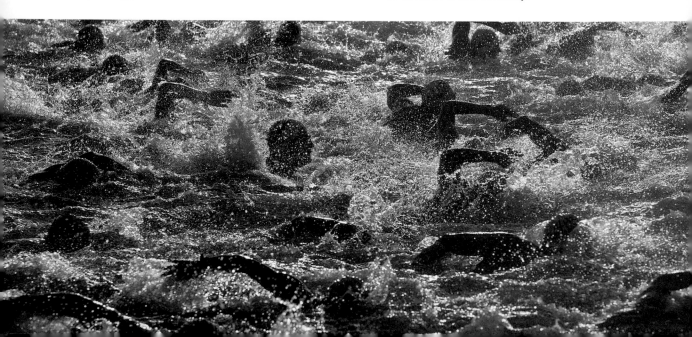

Ex 10.1 Back squat

The back squat is the most common form of the squat exercise and simply refers to the position of the bar. Novice trainers often complain that this feels uncomfortable on their backs and request a foam pad (also known as a sissy pad!) to make it more comfortable. This should be discouraged, not because of macho gym culture but because it is likely to promote poor technique. If the shoulders are pulled back and the chest is made big the upper traps should provide a ridge of muscle for the bar to rest on – even on the skinniest triathlete. If a pad is used the athlete no longer needs to produce this position, and as a result is likely to perform with inferior posture and a looser upper back.

Occasionally an athlete may have such limited mobility in the shoulders that they are unable to hold the bar comfortably in position. In this situation the front squat is a more suitable option. Athletes with particularly long femurs (thigh bone) may also find the back squat difficult. This problem can be countered somewhat by widening the stance or alternatively moving the bar to the front position.

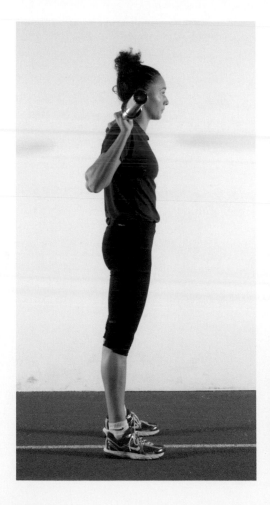
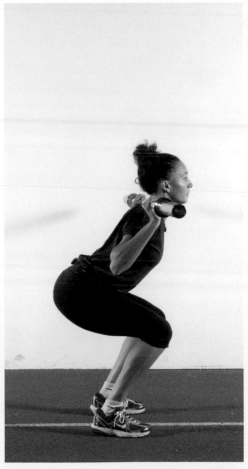

Ex 10.2 Front squat

The front squat is less popular than the back squat, largely due to the fact that it is harder and therefore the weights used tend to be somewhat lighter. However, as already seen, there are a number of situations when the back squat may not be suitable. What is more, the front squat also provides variety and can be used to mix up sessions. The position of the back is generally safer, and it is also more effective for developing back strength.

The biggest obstacle to performing this exercise comes from difficulty holding the bar in the correct position. The bar should be held across the collar bones and almost rest across the wind pipe (*see* below, left). It is crucial that the elbows are kept high throughout the movement in order to prevent the bar pulling the athlete's weight forward at the bottom of the exercise. Many struggle with this, because of a combination of wrist and lat tightness. Ideally you can work through this as the exercise itself will help you to develop mobility in these areas. However if this is too painful or the correct position cannot be achieved then the 'cross arms' technique can be adopted (*see* below, right). Try to avoid using it exclusively, because this will mean that the flexibility required to perform orthodox technique can never be developed.

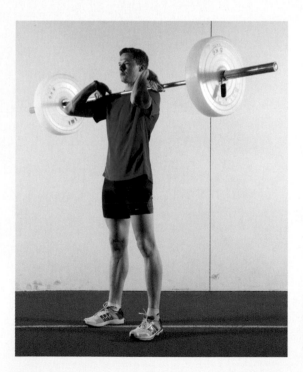
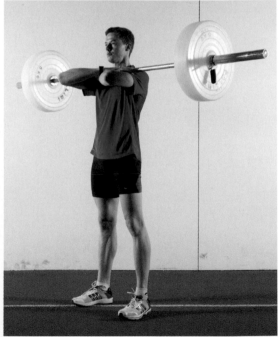

Ex 10.3 Box squats

Both the front and back squats can also be performed as a box squat. This involves sitting the hips backwards to a box or bench and touching lightly (never sitting down fully). This can help in power development because of the need to drive hard off the box; it also provides a good guide to squat depth for consistency. If mobility is a key goal this can be quite motivating – quantifiable improvements can be seen as the boxes and benches get lower and lower.

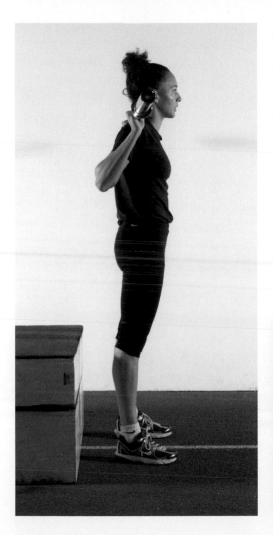
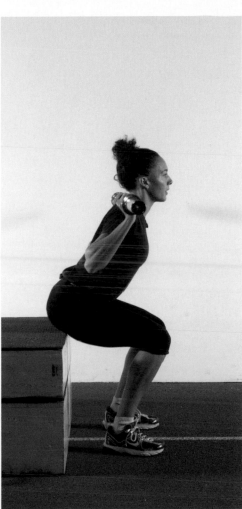

Ex 10.4 Dead lift

Along with the squat, the dead lift is one of the most effective whole body strength exercises at an athlete's disposal. The movements actually appear to be very similar to the naked eye. The biggest difference is that the dead lift is a 'pull' whereas the squat is a 'press'. This means that the dead lift targets the back chain (i.e. lower back, hamstrings and glutes) to a greater extent than the squat, which relies more on the quadriceps on the thigh.

The dead lift is an excellent exercise but should be used with caution. In general an athlete will fail in their technique before they reach the point of true failure (i.e. unable to move the bar). As a result it is very common to see dead lifts performed badly. This will typically come about when either the weight of the bar is too great or the athlete does not have enough mobility to hold form at the bottom of the

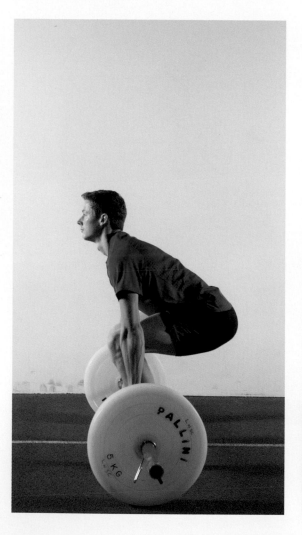
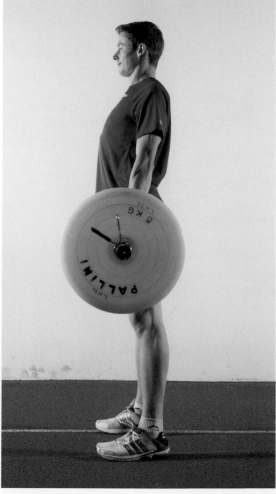

movement. Both of these will result in the lower back rounding. Pulling from this position, even with moderate loads, is very dangerous for the back and should never be accepted. One way in which this can be overcome, other than not overloading the bar, is by raising the height of the bar. The size of the weights discs are completely arbitrary, and so for some people this is not suitable. Therefore if the bar is raised the height of the bar can be changed to suit individual body dimensions. The easiest way to do this is to place weights discs under each end of the bar.

The dead lift has several key coaching points, which are paramount for safe and effective training:

- Keep the back tight and neutral at all times. Any rounding of the back or loss of position should be avoided.
- The start position will vary according to body dimensions, but the shoulders should always be higher than the hips with the feet fully under the bar.
- Start the movement by squeezing the back and lats and by pushing the feet 'through the floor'. This will lead to better technique than simply trying to pull the bar.
- The hips should not be allowed to rise before the chest.
- Keep the bar close to the body at all times.
- Make sure you 'finish' the lift by pressing the hips into the bar and pulling the shoulders back.
- Initiate lowering the bar by sitting the hips backwards. If the movement begins at the knees you will have to swing the bar around the knees, which places it further from the spine and so adds stress.

Single-leg options
While the bilateral exercises are great, many athletes are quick to point out that most sports are performed in a unilateral manner. This is certainly true of all three disciplines in triathlon. During even a very basic movement assessment it quickly becomes clear that many triathletes are very poor when it comes to single-leg stability. This has serious implications for both efficiency of power delivery and injury risk. Therefore some form of single-leg training is a must in any triathlete's S&C regime.

There are a number of different single-leg options, each of which has its own unique characteristics and benefits. Generally these tend to centre around a trade-off between potential for loading (and therefore strength development) and the challenge to stability. Clearly high loading in unstable exercises is not wise. Therefore it is important to establish exactly which of these qualities you wish to target in order to select the appropriate exercise. As outlined earlier in table 5.1, they can broadly be defined as squatting, lunging and stepping patterns. These respectively offer a bias towards strength development, stability or a balance between the two.

Ex 10.5 Bulgarian squat

The Bulgarian squat (also known as rear foot elevated squat) is excellent for developing single-leg strength and provides a good balance of both quad and glute contribution. The fact that the front foot remains in place with weight directly over it provides a 'clamping' effect whereby the knee becomes inherently more stable. This allows it to be loaded to a greater extent than with other exercises.

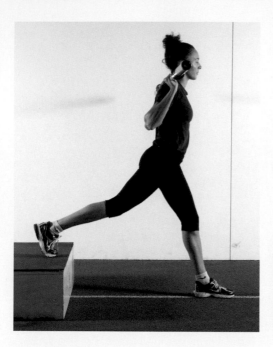 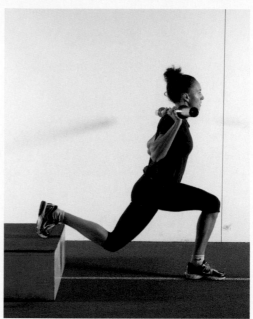

Emphasis
• Single-leg strength

Key points
• Weight should be placed through front foot with knee in line with toes
• Make sure that the foot is placed sufficiently far forwards that the knee does not drift beyond the toes
• Descend to a point whereby the top of the thigh is approximately parallel
• Keep the back tight and chest up
• Do not lock the knee at the top of the movement (remain slightly bent with knee over foot)

Loading
• As a guideline it is achievable to reach a level whereby loads of 75–100% of body weight can be used

Variations
• Although technically a different exercise, the split squat is very similar. Rather than elevating the rear foot the athlete simply adopts a split stance; all other coaching points remain the same

Ex 10.6 Single-leg squat off a box

This is great for demonstrating that you don't always need a barbell to get strong. It is a very challenging movement that uses either body weight or light med balls and is therefore ideal if you travel a lot or do not have access to a gym. The fact that the non-working leg hangs freely allows a great range of movement in the non-working leg. Therefore this often allows athletes to work in ranges that they cannot usually achieve. There is a steep initial learning curve with this movement and after a short time fairly impressive depths can be achieved once the body gets used to these unfamiliar positions.

Emphasis

- Single-leg strength, range of movement and balance

Key points

- Let the free leg hang vertically
- Keep arms out in front to counterbalance
- Keep the back tight and chest up
- Watch for the knee falling inwards (and avoid it)
- Aim to develop a deep position under control

Loading

- Often no additional loading is required and body weight is

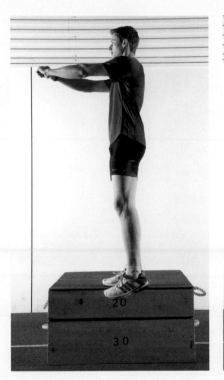
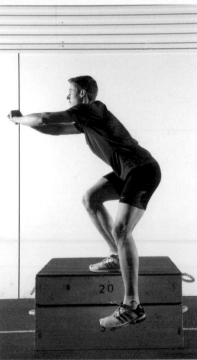

sufficient. However a medicine ball of up to 10kg can be added. This often makes the exercise easier to perform with good technique, because of the counter-balancing effect

Variations

- The pistol is another popular form of single-leg squat (leg held out in front while descending to a box/ bench). While this is also effective the position of holding the leg out in front results in a rounded back and so the off-a-box version is preferable

Ex 10.7 Reverse lunge

Often regarded as no more than a novel derivative of the forward lunge, the reverse lunge is a highly underrated exercise. The more traditional forward version is essentially a force control exercise rather than force generation. For this reason the forward lunge walk is placed in the movement quality conditioning exercises in chapter 9. If knee stability is the athlete's primary focus then I recommend that they utilise this type of work before strengthening. The reverse lunge is a very effective tool for targeting strength in the glutes and hamstrings. The entire lunge series is also an excellent method of developing trunk control during dynamic movements.

Emphasis

- Back chain strength, knee stability, trunk control

Key points

- Step backwards, keeping the weight across the front foot
- Descend to a parallel thigh without the rear knee touching the floor
- Return to the start position by 'pulling through' with the front leg rather than pushing from the rear leg
- Keep the trunk rigid and upright throughout the movement

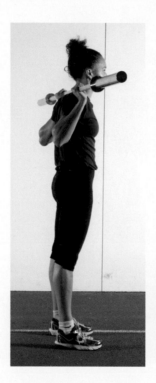
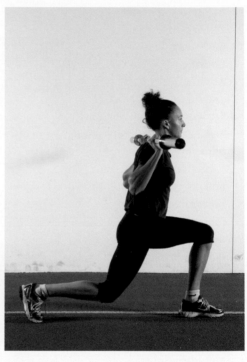

Loading

- Only a light to moderate loading is appropriate with this exercise as one foot comes off the floor: 30kg is generally sufficient for most people

Variations

- There are many possible variations of the lunge (too many to describe in detail). However notable additions include the side lunge and the clock lunge (which uses a combination of forward, reverse and side lunging). Both of these have the relatively unusual feature of working the hips through planes of movement, which is not seen in most gym exercises. Therefore they can be an invaluable addition and help provide more balanced hip stability and mobility

Ex 10.8 Step-ups

Step-ups provide a good balance of both strength development and control. The technique at the start of the movement is crucial as there are many ways to 'cheat', which must be avoided if the exercise is to be fully effective.

Emphasis

- Hip strength, trunk control and knee stability

Key points

- Start with one foot on the box, initiate movement by pushing through the heel
- Avoid leaning the trunk forward or pushing off the back foot to gain momentum at the start of the movement
- Keep the hips high and don't let them sit back during the ascent
- Finish the movement with the knee locked and glute tight with the free leg lifted to a parallel thigh

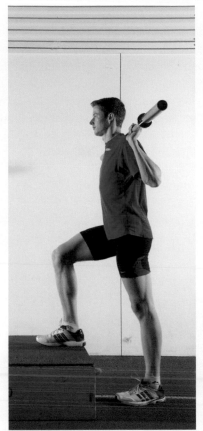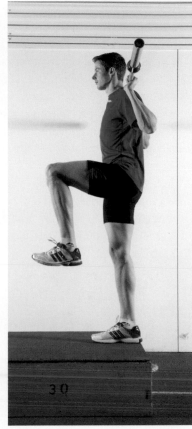

Loading

- Similar to the reverse lunge, a light to moderate loading is appropriate with this exercise as one foot comes off the floor: 0–40kg is generally sufficient for most people

Variations

- The step-up can be tweaked in small ways that make a big difference to the emphasis and outcome. A controlled step with the foot starting on the box is excellent for hip strength and control. Stepping into the box dynamically requires less control because of the momentum; it is more suitable for training power. Also the height of the step can be adapted. A 40cm step is suitable for an average-height athlete (although it can be changed according to height and mobility). The height can be lowered to allow greater loads and thus more emphasis on strength development. Alternatively it can be raised and used with lighter loads for control and mobility to become the focus

Upper body strength

Developing strength in the upper body is important for triathletes for a number of reasons. Apart from more obvious aspects of performance such as the swim stroke and the running arm drive, the upper body also plays a key role in transferring forces around the body and maintaining posture. If either of these is not done effectively then technical performance will suffer. This means that rather than simply building strong arms we need to select exercises that simultaneously work the upper body while holding form through the trunk, etc. Therefore the athlete will often find that their ability to perform these exercises is limited by trunk strength and control rather than sheer brute force. Please note that bench press, bicep curls and any form of machine are notable and deliberate omissions from the triathlete's arsenal!

Ex 10.9 Press-ups

The humble press-up is quite possibly the best upper body exercise ever invented. It offers all the trunk strengthening benefits of the ubiquitous plank plus an excellent method of developing strength through the chest, shoulders and arms.

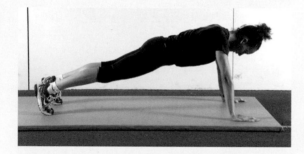 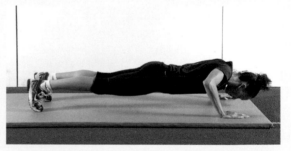

Emphasis
- Chest, shoulders (strength and stability), triceps and trunk

Key points
- Start with and maintain a flat body, lowering to the floor as one unit; do not let the hips sag
- Keep the elbows at approximately 45° to the body
- Good range and a steady tempo are more important than achieving huge numbers of poor-quality repetitions

Loading
- Advanced athletes can add up to a 15kg plate or a weighted vest to advance the exercise.

Placing a plate on the upper or lower back will influence whether it targets the shoulders or trunk

Variations
- There are an almost unlimited number of variations on a press-up and so there really are no excuses for plateauing and sticking with the basic version. Suitable examples include dead press-ups (take hands off the ground at the bottom of each rep) and clap press-ups (good for developing upper body power rather than strength). The use of gymnastic rings of suspension training systems can also dramatically increase the gain in shoulder stability

Ex 10.10 Inverse pulls

One of the detrimental effects of modern daily life on posture is that the muscles of our upper back become long and weak. This in turn leads to even worse posture, poor mechanics and increased risk of shoulder injury. Therefore anything we can do to redress this balance is very welcome. The inverse pull is an ideal tool for this as it works on pulling the shoulder back and opening the chest. Speed of movement is really important if the inverse pull is to be effective – a point that is often missed. The first part of the pull is relatively easy and primarily uses the arms. As the athlete approaches the bar it becomes increasingly harder and the muscles of the upper back come into play more. For this reason many athletes will try to pull hard at the start to generate momentum and make the top half easier. This is obviously flawed as they fail to work the upper back properly, which is the main focus.

Emphasis

- Upper back, biceps and trunk

Key points

- Begin with shoulder-width grip (overhand), body flat and head in neutral (looking forwards and up)
- Shoulders should be pulled back at the start and throughout so that the chest is big and never concave
- Pull up in a controlled manner to a point where the sternum touches the bar without having to arch the back to do so
- As you lower, keep the shoulders pulled back and the chest big

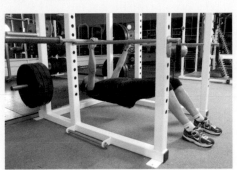

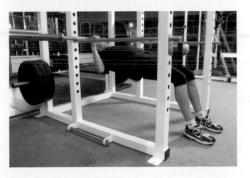

Loading

- Strong athletes may wish to add a weighted vest. Progression beyond this is not needed as control is the key. For a greater strength stimulus athletes should use pull-ups
- As with press-ups, the exercise often needs to be regressed to allow good form. This can be achieved through a couple of variations. The knees can be bent to reduce the weight lifted. Alternatively the height of the bar can be changed. Raising the bar makes the movement easier. It is also possible to have a partner assist you, particularly through the end of the movement where you may be weak

Variations

- Changing the tempo to give an eccentric bias. Try holding the top position for 3–5 seconds and then taking five seconds to descend slowly. You will need to perform fewer reps but will spend much more time working the part of the movement that helps shoulder posture and control
- The use of a suspension training system is useful if the athlete is asymmetric and has issues as a result. This is an effective way of ensuring a balanced development of pulling strength in left versus right

Ex 10.11 Pull-ups

Much like squats, describing pull-ups as simply an upper body exercise does them an injustice. Anyone who has performed both pull-ups and lat pull-downs can attest that there is a lot more to them than simply arms. Unfortunately the exercise can be limited by its difficulty, because many athletes cannot perform a single repetition with appropriate form. Thankfully resistance bands can now be used to gain crucial assistance. The lats play a key role in both the swim stroke and in stabilising the trunk on the bike, so even if the athlete can only perform one or two repetitions it is worth investing time in this movement.

Emphasis

- Upper back and lats, biceps and trunk

Key points

- Select a grip based on target muscles and ability (*see* below)
- Try to keep the shoulders 'set', with the shoulder blades squeezed downwards
- Pull with good control and minimal 'swinging'
- Aim to bring the chest (not the chin) to the bar
- Avoid poking the chin in an attempt to cheat extra height; this will put a strain through the neck and upper back

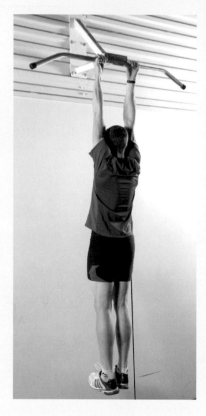
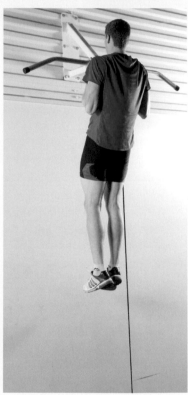

Loading

- The vast majority of athletes should aim to master this exercise through a full range of movement for 8–10 repetitions. Very strong athletes may also use a weighted vest to add variety and overcome plateaux
- Bands can be used to assist the exercise, as can a smaller range. Alternatively, inverse pulls are a good way of building pulling strength in preparation for triathlon

Variations

- There are two main variations of the pull-up, which influence the difficulty and the muscles used: the narrow underhand grip (which is for greater emphasis on arms and is slightly easier); and the wide overhand grip (which targets the upper back and is very difficult)

10.3 Explosive power

Explosive power is the holy grail of most sports. As described in chapter 2, even in endurance sports it is speed that separates the winners from the losers. It can be tempting to leap straight into power work, but this will yield only limited gains because it must be supported by a base of strength. That said, the act of producing a single explosive movement, which represents all of an athlete's capacity in an instant, is a skill that requires much practice. While the likes of sprinters and weightlifters are highly trained at maximal efforts, the nervous system of the endurance athlete is often unfamiliar with such tasks. As a result quite impressive gains can be achieved without any physical change at all – the athlete just becomes more skilled at summoning a greater extent of their capacity. The key to making these gains comes from intent. Every effort must be made to concentrate on producing the absolute most explosive effort possible. Simply going through the motions will be a waste of time.

The exercises in this section are naturally suitable for power development because they involve an acceleration through the movement rather than decelerating as most exercises demand. The most accessible and effective tool is the jump series. Therefore I recommend the athlete focuses on building skills in the jumps rather than using a vast range of different power exercises. When combined with special strength training methods (*see* chapters 8 and 11) these will give an excellent basis for performance enhancement.

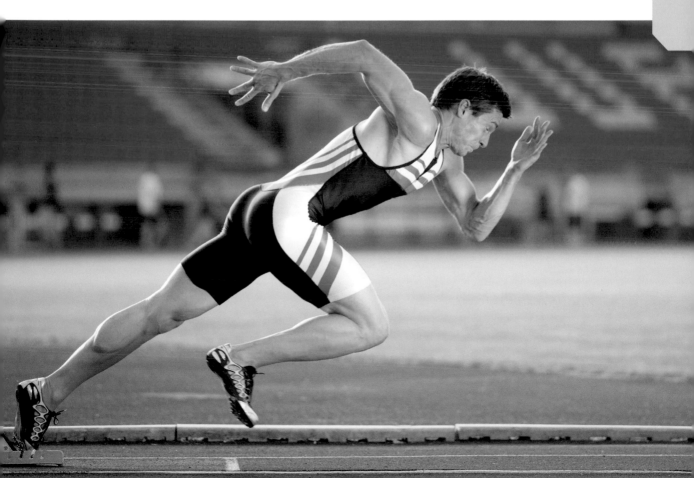

Ex 10.12 Jump series

Jumps are not only the single best movement for power development in triathletes, but they also form a foundation for many other power movements. As well as working as explosively as possible it is also vital to focus on attaining good technique. If the body parts do not work in the correct order the ability to produce and express force will be highly limited. The basis for all jump skills is the counter-movement (CM) jump, which is described below along with key variations.

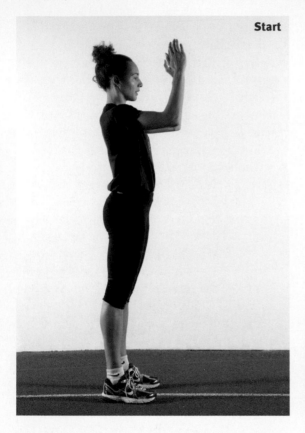

Start

Mid-point

Emphasis
• Whole/lower body power

Key points
• Start with feet about shoulder width apart
• Descend rapidly, keeping the chest up. Be careful not to descend too low; simply dip as you would when aiming to jump as high as possible

• Aim to 'bounce' out of the bottom. The transition between descent and the jump should be as brief as possible
• As you descend make sure the whole of the foot stays in contact with the ground – do not drift on to the toes
• As you jump the movement should flow from the hips to the knees, ankles extending last
• Aim to be fully extended and as tall as possible in the air

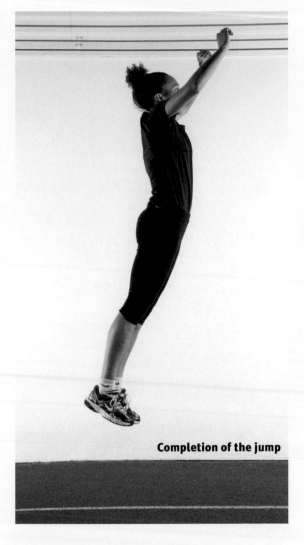

Completion of the jump

Loading

- There is no need to load the counter-movement jump as the greatest power outputs come from jumping with body weight alone
- The movement can be used in a jump squat, although this is a separate exercise rather than an automatic progression

Variations

- A useful variation on the basic jump is a jump to a box. The height of the box can be manipulated by adding/removing weights discs. This helps to quantify training gains and also pushes the athlete on to greater efforts as they work harder to beat previous best jumps
- Jumping to a smaller box and landing straight-legged is another twist that helps to promote a full extension and a taller position in the air
- Rebound jumps are excellent for developing reactive/elastic strength. This involves continuous jumping, with the aim being to land with minimal bending at the hips and knees and to bounce rather than jump. This should mean that time on the floor is kept to an absolute minimum
- Hops are very similar to jumps in terms of the movement and the benefits. The hop requires a little more skill and control but naturally lends itself to the rapid change from descent to jump. Hops can also be performed to a box or in a rebound series

Ex 10.13 Medicine ball toss

Medicine balls (also known as med balls) are naturally suitable for power work and can provide some variety to the jump series. The medicine ball toss is a great whole body exercise that uses a jump-like pattern to direct force into throwing the ball rather than jumping high.

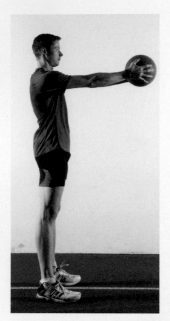
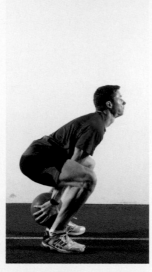
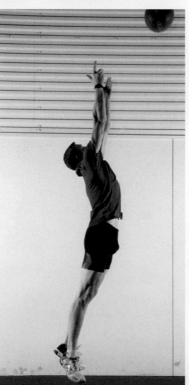

Emphasis

- Whole/lower body power

Key points

- Start with feet about shoulder width apart with the arms held out parallel to the floor and holding the med ball
- The descent is identical to a counter-movement jump. As you bend the legs the arms should naturally lower in rhythm so that they hang vertically at the bottom of the movement
- Explode with the legs, allowing the arms to swing up naturally
- Movement must come from the hips and legs first. If the arms try to throw the ball rather than swing then the power will not be transferred from the legs
- Fully extend the whole body and launch the ball as high as you possibly can

Loading

- If the ball is too heavy technique will suffer. If it is too light the athlete won't be able to develop enough force. Most athletes will work best with a ball of 3–8kg

Variations

- The med ball toss can be adapted to a forward toss or an overhead toss. The difference in training outcome is very minor for the triathlete, and so these are more likely to be used for variety than anything else

Ex 10.14 Medicine ball slam

The medicine ball slam is primarily of interest to those seeking to improve pulling power for the swim. The movement involves a powerful overhead pull in concert with the trunk.

Emphasis
Pulling power

Key points
- The ball is lifted with both hands above the head as the athlete goes up on to their toes
- The ball is powerfully 'slammed' towards the floor keeping the arms long
- Power development begins by contracting the abs (without letting the trunk flex) and the power spreads out from the trunk to the arms (not the other way around)

Loading
- A ball of 4–10kg is generally most suitable for the slam

Variations
- Skilled athletes may be able to perform a single-arm version with a lighter ball

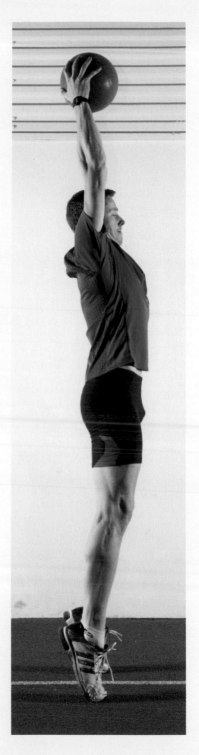

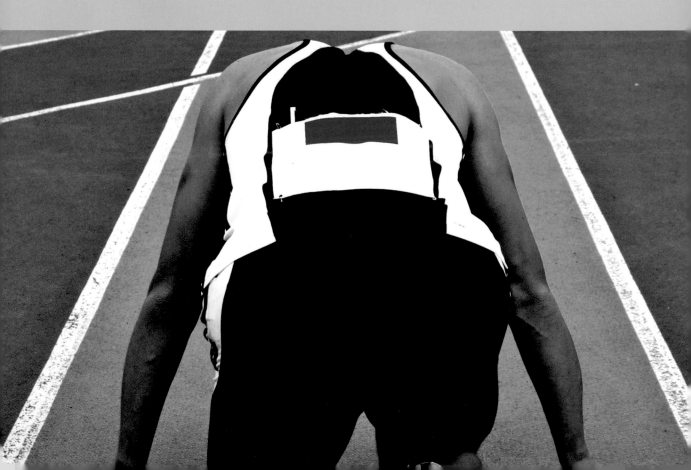

011
specific strength exercises

11.1 Introduction

Specific strength is very much the icing on the cake of strength and conditioning. It is here that many of the foundation qualities that have been developed earlier in the programme are 'moulded' into performance qualities. Unfortunately the eye-catching nature of this work and its obvious relationship with the triathlon disciplines mean that too many athletes are drawn to this work without having established these basic qualities. While a cake with no icing may seem somewhat dull it is still preferable to icing on its own!

An interesting question arises as to who 'owns' this type of work. For the novice who coaches themselves this may not be an issue. For the elite triathlete who has input from both a triathlon coach and an S&C coach it may be less clear. I would suggest it is best left to an individual decision as to who is technically and practically best placed to deliver this training. In an ideal world the two coaches should liaise closely, with programming and delivery being split between both roles.

11.2 Specific swimming strength

Historically coaches have attempted to improve 'swimming strength' through traditional gym exercises, which use similar movements to the swim stroke. This tends to bring about mixed results and in my view is a flawed plan. These types of exercises are generally compromised in terms of force, because the ability to load is sacrificed in favour of stroke replication. This means that the capacity for strength gains is limited. On the other hand, while these movements may appear similar to the swim stroke, variations in load, timing and muscle

recruitment mean that the skill and motor control involved are very different. As a result the transfer at best will be poor and at worst will risk interference with water technique.

I would strongly advocate a philosophy that develops swimming-relevant (rather than swimming-specific) strength in general training. When complemented by the correct work in the pool, this can then begin to transfer into swim strength. Of course this begs the question: 'What is the correct work in the pool to achieve this transfer?' The answer lies in the following types of work, which can be used for special swimming strength:

- Sprint efforts
- Bungee/tethered resisted swims
- Bungee/tethered assisted swims
- Float kicking exercises
- Float arm exercises

Sprint efforts

Possibly the best form of special strength training for the swim component of a triathlon is performing sprint efforts. If strength training is about working appropriate movements at a greater intensity than usually experienced then this fits precisely. In order to make sure that the movement is as close as possible to 'normal swimming' and that there is no negative transfer of poor technique every effort should be made not to change the stroke. The only other issue that must be considered when doing sprints is the sets, reps, distances and recovery. The volume of work should not be so high that a good intensity cannot be maintained, but it also needs to be enough to achieve a training effect. Therefore this will be somewhat individual. However a typical block of strength work may consist of 50-metres all-out efforts with a 1:2 work:rest ratio.

A decision also needs to be made as to how 'pure' the work will be. Many triathletes will already use repeated sprints with limited recovery as part of a high-intensity fitness session. This may still have a strengthening effect but is very much a hybrid strength/fitness session. The smart coach or athlete will use a combination of pure strength sessions (or blocks within a session) and hybrid work to provide variety and match the aims of the particular phase of training.

Bungee/tethered resisted and assisted swims

Resisted and assisted swims have always been popular tools among swim coaches. This can be achieved through tether ropes, bungee cords or water jet pools. Resisted swimming enables the swimmer to develop a greater ability to produce propulsive force, whereas assisted swimming develops stroke rate. Like many areas of coaching though this remains an area of much debate. Both of these methods have been found to have positive effects on swim performance. The evidence for this is both anecdotal from coaches and scientific through controlled studies. Despite this others still argue that these methods have detrimental effects on technique when being performed. On balance I would suggest that even though technique may suffer during these efforts it seems that the outcome is still faster swimming. On that basis it is worth using. However it is probably best to avoid this work if the athlete's technique is poor already, if they have recently made technical changes or at times close to competition.

Float kicking and float arm exercises

Similar arguments can be made when using a float to place a specific emphasis on the arm action or the kick. These are often used to develop technique and so it is entirely possible to

maintain form while developing propulsion power. Once again the key here is to make sure that the goal of the session is clear (i.e., strength, technique, conditioning, etc.). Just doing some float exercises will achieve little unless the physical intensity and mental focus are matched to the goal.

11.3 Specific cycling strength

When we talk of cycling strength we often end up on dangerous ground. The intensities we work at and the durations that they can be sustained for mean that what we actually develop are strength endurance or power. Even a very short hill of 60 seconds means we have drifted into endurance. When riders talk about doing a 60-minute strength ride it is clear that pure strength is not being developed. Similarly even short efforts of several seconds in a high gear are not true strength. Although the intensity is high and the duration is short the force generated is only moderate in comparison with true strength training. (Don't get confused between force and power. The highest forces occur at slow speeds so if we are moving quickly we will have high power but moderate force.) All of this is not cited to denigrate the importance of bike work; it simply means that it must be used in conjunction with other methods that will develop force-generating abilities to lay a platform for this work.

Essentially cycle-specific strength sessions consist of much shorter efforts than normal, working against a tough resistance with good recovery time. This increase in resistance can come either from hills or cranking up the gears (or a combination of the two). Personally I would advocate doing this type of work predominantly on a stationary bike. This will allow the athlete to precisely plan and monitor the resistance used

Table 11.1	Cycling-specific strength options			
Session	**Target**	**Setting**	**Duration**	**Recovery**
Power sprints	Power	Indoor bike with high gear	8–20 secs	1:10
Hills	Strength endurance	Steep hill or indoor high resistance	3–5 mins	1:1
Big gear efforts	Power endurance	Indoor or outdoor with high gear	30–90 secs	1:2

rather than relying on the local geography. It is also useful for measuring small improvements and is safe as the athlete can get their head down without fear of traffic! Having said that, there is a lot to be said for the motivational benefits of taking on a vicious hill – particularly in competition with training partners.

There are lots of different permutations for these types of workout. Table 11.1 gives a starting point for defining the types of session the athlete should do and how they might look.

11.4 Specific running strength

Specific strength for running is a whole different ball game when compared to the other two disciplines of triathlon. Swimming involves generating propulsion to overcome resistance through the water, while in cycling the athlete pushes against the resistance of the crank and the significant drag factor caused by air flow. In both sports resistance increases with speed. The same cannot be said of running. Here the main resistance to overcome is gravity, which remains constant throughout. As a result much, although not all, specific strength for running is concerned with the motor control or postural strength required to hold good form. However this is not the only form of specific work. We can also use plyometrics and high-intensity running to improve reactive/elastic strength and make running more efficient. The concept and methods of using fast running and sprints for enhancing running mechanics are discussed in chapter 6.

Exercises to improve technique

People don't run with poor technique because they haven't been shown what to do. Poor running technique comes about through poor conditioning and poor control (*see* chapter 6). Gym work will effectively target conditioning, but postural control is highly specific. The running drills below are the most effective method of improving this control. There is also a conditioning effect, which will give the body the ability to hold form. The intensity of the exercises is very low, so there must be a very strong mental focus on technique.

The devil is truly in the detail with these exercises. It is for this reason that I have strongly criticised magazine articles that use still photos. Therefore I would urge you to seek expert coaching where possible seek expert coaching. This will enable you to get the most from the drills and perform them with confidence.

Ex 11.1 A-march

The A-march is a fairly basic drill but can have big effects. Most runners have a style that coaches describe as 'sitting down'. This means that the hips are set back and the knee is quite flexed. This tends to lead to longer ground contact times and less efficient running.

Emphasis
- Postural control

Typical volume
- 10–30 metres with walk back recovery
- 3–6 reps per session

Key points
- The focus of the A-march is to squeeze the glute of the standing leg to get the hips as high as possible
- Try to be as tall as possible; imagine you have a fish hook lifting your belly button
- Lift the chest without leaning backwards
- Lift the knee of the free leg without straining and keep the toes pulled up towards the shin

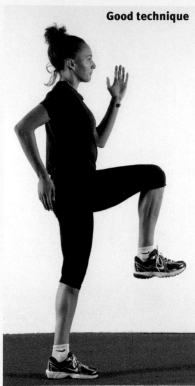

Good technique

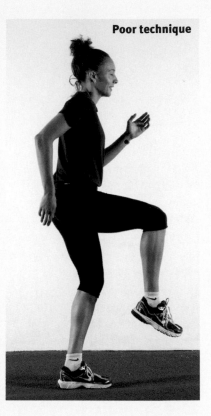

Poor technique

Variations/Progressions
- This can be progressed into increasingly more dynamic versions of the movement, which are more challenging to control, for example, an A-skip or a 'jogging' knee lift drill. These can be combined with strides (form running over 30–50 metres), which greatly help to transfer the drill into 'real running'. However do not be tempted to progress until you have mastered the march with ease

Ex 11.2 Skipping

This is a very simple exercise, but there are some key benefits to be gained from it. A basic skip can help to promote some key shapes that are important for good running mechanics. This includes a 'hip–knee–toe' lifting of the thigh (*see* chapter 6), good tall posture and a positive arm drive. Furthermore skipping also helps to develop ankle stiffness (not to be confused with stiff ankles). This is critical for elastic efficiency. There is even the possibility of power development as progressions move towards the power skip.

Emphasis
- Running mechanics, ankle stiffness and postural control

Typical volume
- 20–40 metres with walk back recovery
- 150–200 metres total work per session

Key points
- For the basic skip start nice and easy and loose; let the arms swing freely and naturally
- Keep the contacts on the ground short and sharp rather than heavy and long. Look to be bouncy rather than land and jump

Variations
- The basic skip is a good warm-up drill, which can be progressed into a more intense version. As the intensity increases focus on driving the high upwards to create greater lift. This should produce a greater time in the air without sacrificing time on the floor (i.e., long hang time with very short contact time). Look to hold a strong position in the air and anticipate the landing, rather than waiting then reacting

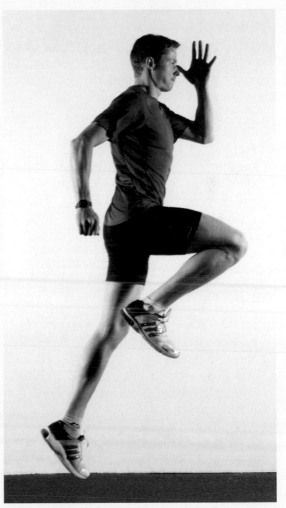

Ex 11.3 Hurdle drills

Hurdle drills have long been a staple in the training of track and field athletes from all events. Fear not though. These do not involve sprinting towards a high barrier, but instead use hurdles as obstacles to walk or skip through. The main benefits of these drills are excellent postural control and mobility. More advanced skipping versions can also improve rhythm and stiffness.

There is one small problem though, in that full-sized hurdles require a level of mobility that is beyond many. Fortunately smaller hurdles, which are intended purely for these drills, are now available. Nevertheless I have still seen many elite sports people performing these drills with terrible posture as the hurdle is too high. Obviously practising postural control in poor postures is not what we are looking for. Therefore I would suggest that the athlete uses any object of a height that they can cope with or even just an imaginary hurdle. There are literally hundreds of variations of these exercises, but we will focus on the basic hurdle walk-through, which is a great method of building strength and mobility through the hips.

Emphasis
- Hip strength and mobility, postural control

Typical volume
- 6 hurdles per set
- 3–5 sets per session

Key points
- Lift the lead knee, keeping the spine tall (don't let your back round) and your hips high (squeeze the standing glute and keep the knee locked)
- Step over the hurdle keeping the shin hanging vertically and the foot pulled up towards the shin
- The trail leg comes over by opening out the thigh so that the inner thigh faces forwards
- This is then lifted over and round without losing any posture through the trunk

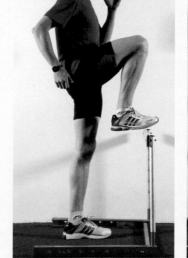
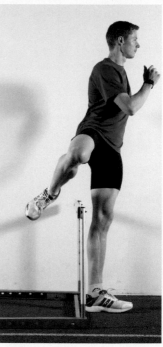

Variations
- As mobility progresses the height of the hurdle/barrier can gradually be increased
- Some useful variations include holding the arms out to the side or holding a light ball above the head
- Other typical drills that can be useful include lateral leg swings and high knees down the side of the hurdles

Ex 11.4 No arms running

This one is a little left-field but I have decided to include it as I have had such good results when working with athletes who are developing basic running skills. I cannot take credit for this exercise as the idea was introduced to me by the running mechanics expert Frans Bosch. His idea is very simple in that the athlete simply runs at close to maximum effort, but without using their arms. This can be done in several ways including the athlete wrapping their arms around themselves or holding a light stick across their shoulders, as in a back squat. The effect is quite stark: all of a sudden the athlete is forced to bring the trail leg through far quicker in order to keep balanced. This in turn has further implications, with much less rotation to control and a taller more athletic-looking posture. The great thing about no arms running is that it requires no coaching – the aim is for the athlete's body to 'learn' how to run rather than their mind. This makes the exercise ideal for triathletes who do not have regular access to expert supervision.

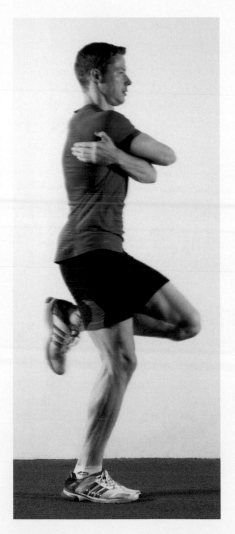

Emphasis
• Running mechanics

Typical volume
• 5–8 runs of approximately 50 metres

Key points
• Run at a pace hard enough to force you to have to drive the knees forwards
• Concentrate on how the body 'feels' running this way and then replicate this feeling during normal runs (alternate drill and normal running)
• Focus on these feelings rather than thinking about technique

Variations
• Use either arms wrapped around the chest or a bar/stick across the shoulders

index

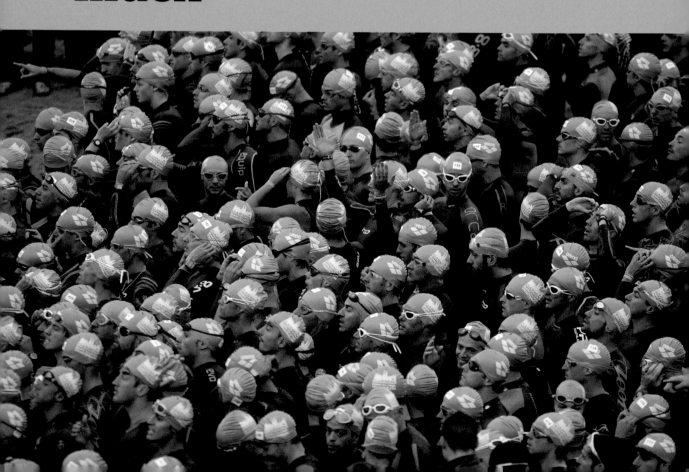